Hospital Turnarounds

Lessons in Leadership

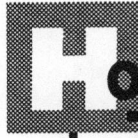

Hospital Turnarounds

Lessons in Leadership

Terence F. Moore and
Earl A. Simendinger

BeardBooks

Washington, DC

Library of Congress Cataloging-in-Publication Data

Hospital turnarounds : lessons in leadership / [edited by] Terence F. Moore
    and Earl A. Simendinger.
        p.   cm.
    Originally published: Ann Arbor, Mich. : Health Administration Press, c1993.
    Includes bibliographical references and index.
    1. Hospitals—United States—Business management—Case studies.
2. Hospitals—United States—Administration—Case studies.
I. Moore, Terence F.   II. Simendinger, Earl A.
[RA971.3.H67   1999]
362.1'1'068—dc21   99-13210
                                                        CIP

Printed in the United States of America

To Carleen K. Moore,
Albert A. Moore, and
Diana White

CONTENTS

ACKNOWLEDGMENTS

Our deepest thanks to Peggy Oliver, administrative assistant, MidMichigan Regional Health System, for her excellence.

Our thanks to Daphne Grew, Director, Health Administration Press, Edward Kobrinski, Acquisitions Editor, and the entire staff of Health Administration Press, for their efforts. Anthony Kovner also assisted greatly in reviewing the initial manuscript.

Lastly, our sincere thanks to those who authored or coauthored the chapters contained herein. Every one of them is a top professional.

ACKNOWLEDGMENTS

INTRODUCTION

Terence F. Moore and Earl A. Simendinger

Almost all hospitals and other health care institutions are going through a period of financial duress that is unprecedented in recent history. The number of hospitals that have closed is at an all time high, and many more might close within the next few years.

That more hospitals have not closed to date is due in large part to a select group of health care executives who have led their institutions from potentially disastrous situations to financial viability. These turnaround artists are often the unsung heroes of their institutions and represent the highest standards of excellence of health care professionals. Their collective excellence has saved millions of dollars in health care expenditures and saved numerous institutions from closing, thereby providing better accessibility while often increasing the overall quality of the care that is being provided. If they were in the military, these individuals would be the highly decorated battalion and brigade commanders who win numerous battles, often against overwhelming odds.

The various chapters in this book were written by such men and women. Through a number of sources, we located 14 health care executives in the United States who have achieved truly remarkable financial turnarounds in their institutions. Some already have national reputations; all should have. Some oversee hospitals as small as 42 beds, and some run major health care systems. They represent most geographic areas in the United States. Their stories describe the techniques, tactics, and politics of financially turning around health care organizations. The lessons in this book apply not only to those who are faced with turning around a potentially financially disastrous situation but to all those who are responsible for improving the financial altitude of their institutions—that includes most health care executives at all levels.

For our purposes, we have defined a turnaround as a situation in which the health care facility or system significantly improved its financial operating margins, usually within two years but sometimes within one year. In some cases, the hospital went from a loss position to a slight profit. In some situations, the hospital's profitability showed a dramatic and sustained increase over three or four years.

To date, only one book has been published about hospital turnarounds: *Managing a Hospital Turnaround: From Crisis to Profitability in Three Challenging Years,* by Michael Rindler.[1] However, turnarounds in other industries have been extensively researched and well documented for several decades. The last chapter describes the results of some of that research and how it compares with the turnarounds described by the authors of this book. From the descriptions of various turnarounds, it becomes apparent that the general stages of a turnaround in hospitals are similar to those in other industries. Rindler's book provides an excellent overview of one turnaround in one midsize hospital. Our intent was to document a number of turnarounds and then summarize the key lessons to be learned from these summaries for present day and future health care leaders.

Of the numerous typologies that exist for organizational turnarounds, the one that appears most applicable to health care organizations has five stages. The first of these stages is the taking hold stage, in which there is much learning and action. When the situation is understood, the second stage begins. This is the emergence stage, in which the chief executive officer (CEO) and the management team immerse themselves in running the organization in a more formalized fashion. The third stage, the reshaping stage, is the period of greatest activity. The most significant downsizing activities usually occur during this stage. The fourth stage is the consolidation stage, which is usually a period of little change. The last stage, the refinement stage, involves the fine tuning of the organization and must be ongoing if a turnaround is to be sustained. An example is the institution of total quality management programs by health care institutions throughout the United States. These programs are a tool for maximizing the organization's potential and are important to the refinement stage. Chapter 12 discusses how theses stages were manifested in the turnarounds described in Chapters 1 through 11.

We have asked each author or coauthor to document the role of the various publics in the turnaround. What was the role of the board, the role of the medical staff, the role of the management team, and the role of volunteers? Some wrote in greater detail about some of these publics than others. The last chapter summarizes the role of each of these various publics with particular attention to the role of the management team. In addition, we have summarized the key mistakes made in turnarounds, as described by the authors and other experts.

A turnaround is most often the result of increased revenues and decreased expenses. Some of the authors focused on increasing revenues to improve the operating margins of their organizations, and some focused almost exclusively on reducing expenses. However, to maximize the potential of a turnaround necessitates that executives focus on both reducing expenses and increasing revenues. The authors orchestrated their turnarounds in slightly different ways.

Lastly, some of the factors that are necessary to prevent organizational decline or organizational burnout are outlined. The need for upward communication, fluidity of organizational structure, a reduction of unnecessary bureaucratic rules and policies, and ambitious yet realistic goals and objectives are described. Organizational burnout occurs when the sum of an organization's actual output is decreasing over time when compared to its potential output. To reduce this gap, the gap between an organization's potential output and its actual output, is the challenge of executives in any organizational setting.

Almost anyone can downsize an organization. The art is to minimize the trauma while maximizing the organization's potential. A complicating factor is that the turnaround artist must also avoid losing his or her job in the process. This book does not attempt to analyze the difference between those executives who turned around their organizations and were forced to leave and those executives who did not lose their jobs. Although several of the authors have moved from the institutions they turned around (two of them have even moved twice, each time to a progressively better position), none of them were forced by their boards to leave.

We hope that this book will be a valuable resource for all health care professionals who are charged with the survival and improvement of their institutions and therefore enhance their own professional survival.

Note

1. M. Rindler, *Managing a Hospital Turnaround: From Crisis to Profitability in Three Challenging Years* (Chicago: Pluribus Press, Inc., 1987).

1

LEADERSHIP TRANSITION AND DIAGNOSIS IN A HOSPITAL TURNAROUND: A CONTRAST IN LEADERSHIP APPROACHES

R. Timothy Stack

Editors' Note: This chapter was chosen as the first chapter because it focuses on the first phase (the diagnostic phase) of a hospital turnaround. The methods used to assess the true nature of a health care organization, its problems and potentials, are outlined. The approach right before a new CEO arrives and the communication process used once the executive has arrived are also described. The chapter also describes various turnaround models from the literature that the turnaround leader can adapt. It serves as a basis for comparison in the following chapters when the diagnostic phase of a turnaround is discussed.

In the short span of my career as a health care executive, the industry has progressed from the halcyon period of cost reimbursement through the frenetic phase of corporate reorganization and diversification to our current period of prospective payment compression and in some cases hospital failures. Decreased utilization, reduced reimbursement, discounts, charity care, and bad debt are taking their toll. Inflation, technology, unions, professional staff shortages, and other factors drive up costs despite efforts to control them. Consequently, ordinary belt tightening is no longer a viable option for many hospitals. Hospital closures are becoming commonplace, and predictions call for more closures.

Into this milieu has come a new specialist among the ranks of health care executives: the turnaround expert. Previously unheard of in health

5

care, this new breed of health care executive is rare at this point. If predictions of additional difficult times ahead hold true for the health care industry, however, the turnaround specialist might become commonplace.

This chapter highlights the role of the CEO in a health care organization in which a corporate turnaround either is imminent or needs to be forestalled. The material is based on a composite of personal experiences and on research as well as interviews undertaken in preparation of my fellowship project for the American College of Healthcare Executives.

The Situation Before and After Turnaround

Before describing the diagnostic process, phases of the turnaround process, factors affecting the process, and insights gained in carrying out turnarounds, it is useful to provide an overview.

Situation Before the Turnaround

The board and leadership are often demoralized, and employees are fearful, anxious about their jobs, and largely unproductive. Cash flow is usually so low that borrowing is necessary to meet the payroll. The medical staff is upset to the point of withholding admissions or using alternative hospitals if they are available. Effective policies and systems are nonexistent or are not being used. The environment is tense, and the myriad of complex problems seems unsolvable. But the stereotypical situation just described is not always the case.

In contrast, in a near-turnaround situation, the organization might appear ordinary on the surface. The appearance of business as usual masks the deep underlying problems that threaten the financial viability of the organization. No one speaks of the major problems. Denial of reality is the essence of this situation.

Either one of these two contrasting situations might exist in the health care organization. I have personally experienced both. Both are equally threatening to the hospital. Both are equally challenging to the turnaround leader.

These two dissimilar turnaround situations are usually faced using one of two contrasting approaches. One approach could be characterized as an intuitive approach based largely on well developed instincts. The other approach is much more systematic and based on both prior hands-on experience and lessons learned from the business literature on corporate turnaround. Both approaches can work. The lesson of this chapter, however, is that the more systematic approach that uses techniques and knowledge in the literature on turnarounds is preferred. Turnaround success will come a lot easier if executives use previously developed models to visualize the process and apply proven techniques from the literature to carry it out.

The following are common elements of difficulty found in hospitals facing a turnaround or near turnaround:

1. The governing board is too large, its composition is inappropriate to the situation, its actions are passive rather than proactive, and board development is lacking.
2. The medical staff leadership is weak, uncommitted to the hospital, and focused on opposing goals rather than mutual goals.
3. Executive management is ineffective in fulfilling both its operational and strategic management responsibilities.
4. There are too many middle managers, so professionals capable of autonomy are overmanaged.
5. The corporate structure is too tall and top heavy with staff.
6. Operational problems are being overlooked because it is more exciting to pursue the latest fad.
7. Emphasis is placed on a long-range planning process rather than on actively managing today's strategic issues.

More generally, the organization might be suffering from over-expansion, excessive leverage, too much diversification, too little utilization, unfavorable reimbursement contracts, or simply mismanagement. Any or all of these conditions might have contributed to the need for turnaround actions.

The bleak situation just described was not found in my most recent experience and might not be found in every case, but many of these elements are encountered in a turnaround situation.

Situation After the Turnaround

If the turnaround plan contained carefully prepared, reasonable performance targets, one might declare success when these turnaround targets have been met. But success can be short lived if the sustaining actions that underlie these performance measures have not been satisfactorily accomplished. It is one thing to achieve a short-run operating success and quite another to ensure the long-term stability, viability, and growth of the organization.

The situation following my most recent near-turnaround effort is presently favorable, especially the operational indicators. Expenses have been dramatically reduced. Operating margins have exceeded targets, and quality indicators are up to standards.

Aside from the operating indicators, the organization has now returned to a period of stability. A new, much leaner organizational structure is in place. All executive positions are filled with talented team players. A new mission and corporate vision statement have been developed. A grand strategy has been decided, and various business plans are completed or underway. The principal goals now being pursued are a return to growth and continued stability. The challenges of this stage in a turnaround are addressed below.

Transition

Assuming that the turnaround executive has just taken the position of CEO (and this is almost always the case), the first important action in the turnaround process begins before the new executive actually arrives. This three-step preliminary transition process starts with the development of a transition plan, includes a macrolevel analysis of the organization, and culminates with the preparation of the initial turnaround plan.

Prearrival Transition Plan

Many CEOs prefer to approach a new position informally by simply arriving at the office to begin work without having done any significant preparation before arrival. They then informally begin to learn about the organization, usually through applying their skills gained through prior experience. There are two major drawbacks of this approach. The learning time is lengthy and the lack of a structured evaluation increases the likelihood that the new CEO might miss important areas during this early stage.

In a turnaround or near turnaround, this slow-going, informal, intuitive approach is not likely to be effective. There just is not enough time. When the organization is hemorrhaging cash, a more formal approach to transition is indicated. A well-written transition plan can serve this purpose.

The preparation and execution of a transition plan to ensure an orderly, productive, and quick transition of the new chief executive into the organization is highly recommended. There are three major objectives in preparing a transition plan: (1) to ensure proper introductions to and initial rapport with key stakeholder's of the organization, (2) to saturate the CEO with relevant data and supporting information on the organization, and (3) to expedite a general initial evaluation of the corporation to pinpoint major areas that need immediate attention while a turnaround plan is being prepared.

Before actually arriving at the new position, the newly appointed CEO should contact the organization to (1) arrange for the collection and availability of materials to be reviewed either before arrival or immediately on arrival; (2) appoint a transition task force to facilitate the process; (3) have the executive suite staff prearrange individual in-depth interviews with members of the senior executive group, the chair of the board, and the chief of the medical staff; and (4) have the executive suite staff set up briefings by the heads of all major subsidiary organizations as well as the heads of all major functional areas within the organization.

Guidelines regarding materials the CEO wishes to review should be clearly communicated to the executive suite staff and to the transition task force. As an example, such guidelines might include the following: (1) all lengthy written material is to have an executive summary attached; (2) no raw data (e.g., computer printouts) will be accepted without an attached analysis and summary; (3) the origin of information is to be clearly marked with the name, title, and telephone number of the preparer; (4) each problem or issue raised is to be accompanied by a brief report of actions previously taken as well as possible alternatives for further action; and (5) where possible, information is to be summarized in a matrix format. Without such advance guidelines, the CEO is likely to get mountains of raw data and reams of unanalyzed information.

A decision must also be made regarding what to have sent in advance and what is to be waiting in the office. Exhibit 1.1 presents examples of material to be reviewed before arrival and immediately on arrival.

Having arranged for the collection and availability of relevant material, the next task to be completed before arrival at the new organization is to establish a transition task force. In establishing this task force, it is important to clearly communicate to both the chair and members the purpose, scope of responsibility, and specific objectives to be accomplished. Exhibit 1.2 is an actual charge to an ad hoc task force appointed to facilitate the transition of an incoming chief executive.

Exhibit 1.1   Chief Executive Officer Transition Review Materials

Prearrival Review
1. Corporate legal documents (charter, bylaws)
2. Medical staff bylaws, rules, and regulations
3. Mission, vision, and guiding principles statements
4. Strategic plan
5. Operating plan (goals, budgets, etc.)
6. Current operating reports (summarized)
7. Financial ratio analysis (current and past three years)
8. Business plans (subsidiaries, product lines, etc.)
9. JCAHO report (summarized)
10. Pending and recently approved certificates of need
11. Pending litigation
12. Profile of board members
13. Profile of medical staff leaders
14. Profile of top 20 medical staff admitters
15. Resumes of executives
16. Executive salaries, benefits, and perquisites
17. Position description of executives

Postarrival Review
1. Board minutes
2. Medical staff minutes
3. Minutes of board committees
4. Minutes of medical staff committees
5. Minutes of administrative committees
6. Summary report of external agency evaluations
7. Summary report of internal auditor reports
8. Summary report of medical staff discipline cases
9. Existing union contracts
10. Contracts with external organizations
11. Managed care contracts
12. Contracts with physicians
13. Interorganizational contracts
14. Summary of consultants retained (present and past three years)
15. Administrative policies

A third important task for the CEO before arrival is to have the executive suite staff set up in-depth interviews as previously mentioned. While most new chief executives would do this, the two important points are that (1) the interviews should be done immediately on arrival and thus should be prearranged and (2) the interviews should be structured for optimum benefit rather than being casual. Again time is the essence. See Exhibit 1.3 for key excerpts from a senior executive questionnaire previously tested and proved effective.[1]

A fourth and final task to be arranged in advance is the planning and scheduling of briefings for the new CEO. Briefing content decisions are usually handled best by the transition task force. At a minimum, each briefing should contain (1) a summary description of the subject subsidiary organization or function; (2) a summary of indicators of recent performance; (3) organizational structure; (4) known problems, issues, strengths, weaknesses, opportunities, and threats; and (5) a brief summary of what is presently being done to improve overall performance.

Exhibit 1.2   Charge to Chief Executive Officer Transition Task Force

---

1. Prepare a list of the top 20 organizational stakeholders with greatest influence.
2. Prepare a list of the top 20 problems and issues, with available options as appropriate.
3. Prepare a summary of the organization's strengths, weaknesses, opportunities, risks, and threats.
4. Prepare a summary of the current local and state political climate and issues relevant to the organization.
5. Prepare a list of the organization's sacred cows and comment on each.
6. Supervise the preparation of materials to be gathered for review by the CEO.
7. Supervise the preparation of the briefings to be presented to the CEO on arrival.
8. Be available to the CEO on arrival for one or more meetings as needed.
9. Recommend to the incoming CEO any actions or procedures that will facilitate transition into the organization.

Exhibit 1.3 Chief Executive Officer's Structured Interview with Executives

---

1. What are the duties and responsibilities of your primary position and what proportion of time do you devote to each?
2. What additional duties, responsibilities, and special projects do you have?
3. What specific parameters and standards is your performance evaluated by or should it be evaluated by?
4. What additional resources or authority do you need to effectively fulfill your duties and responsibilities?
5. What functions do you perform that should be performed by others? Specify who the others are.
6. What functions are not presently assigned to you that should be assigned to you?
7. What functions or major tasks within the organization are being duplicated unnecessarily?
8. What functions or major tasks within the organization are not being accomplished?
9. What hampers you in the performance of your duties and responsibilities?
10. What facilitates the effective performance of your duties and responsibilities?
11. What committees or meetings could be eliminated, consolidated, or held less frequently without an untoward impact?
12. If you were CEO, what major changes would you initiate that would likely make the organization more efficient or effective?
13. In what specific ways can the board better support executive managers in fulfilling their duties and responsibilities?
14. In what specific ways can the medical staff better support executive managers in fulfilling their duties and responsibilities?
15. In what specific ways can executive managers better support the board in fulfilling its governance responsibilities?
16. In what specific ways can executive managers better support the medical staff in fulfilling its responsibilities?

Postarrival Actions

When arrangements for review materials, the task force, interviews with key individuals, and briefings have been completed, the CEO is ready to arrive and begin work. The first challenge is to approach the tasks of saturating himself or herself with relevant information and gaining rapport with key stakeholders of the organization. The usual process would be (1) to study thoroughly all material furnished before arriving at the new position; (2) to set aside time during the first two or three days after arrival to review material not mailed in advance; (3) to interview key individuals as previously arranged; (4) to attend prearranged briefings; and (5) to meet with the entire transition task force to clarify or verify initial insights and discuss the preparation of a turnaround plan.

As a result of carrying out a well-thought-out transition plan, it usually becomes obvious that a number of major problems exist if the organization is in a turnaround or near-turnaround situation. These problems might range from a lack of overall operating structure and systems to specific problems in finance, human resources, material, information systems, contracts, and other operational areas. A clear vision of the organization's future and of strategic management is also likely to be lacking. For these reasons, a more detailed diagnostic process must usually follow the CEO's transition into the organization.

Diagnostic Process

When the prearrival and postarrival transition has been completed, attention can then be turned to diagnosis of the major problems of the ailing organization. To adequately understand the organization's problems and to prepare to resolve them is a three-step process. First, it is necessary to have a conceptual understanding and framework. This means developing a clear mental picture of what is involved in the turnaround process and especially what the impact of this process will be on the organization and its people. With a clear conceptual framework in mind, an evaluation plan can then be prepared and implemented to find, classify, and prioritize the organization's problems. Finally, a turnaround plan can be prepared and initiated. A conceptual framework, an evaluation plan, and a formal turnaround plan are three important elements of the diagnostic phase of a turnaround.

Conceptual Framework

As used in this context, a conceptual framework is simply a structured way of mentally viewing the turnaround. The turnaround leader must form a mental image of the process. Forming this mental picture of what is about to happen is important for several reasons: (1) the image provides a structure around which actual plans and actions can be developed, (2) the image provides a framework for mentally rehearsing the events to come to improve the probability of success and to anticipate potential problems in the process, (3) the conceptual framework facilitates communication as well as understanding of the process throughout the organization by giving everyone involved a common focal point, and (4) the conceptual framework serves as a base line for keeping the evaluation and turnaround processes on track.

Three models from the literature have proved most useful in developing a conceptual framework. First, a model developed by Bibeault presents an excellent mental image of the five stages in a turnaround.[2] A less conceptual but very useful model by Sloma presents, in a flowchart, 13 detailed action steps that are usually taken in turnarounds.[3] Finally, an excellent model by Bridges addresses the human impact of the transition from the old organization to the new.[4] Each of these three models has been applied successfully in hospital turnarounds.

Diagnostic Tools

Before addressing diagnostic tools, the importance of using insights gained during the transition process outlined above and the value of using the three conceptual models described above must be stressed. Insights from these two sources makes the use of diagnostic tools much more productive.

Specific descriptions of various quantitative methods, financial ratios, and similar diagnostic tools are commonly available and thus are not addressed. There is no single best process to follow in the initial evaluation in a turnaround. It would be a mistake to simply select a process and force fit it to the particular situation at hand. Each turnaround or near turnaround is unique in many respects. My experiences indicate that a combination or synthesis of widely used evaluative approaches tailored to the specific situation works best. Among the most useful of these overall approaches are the following:

1. Goldstick's ABC classifications of elements that affect the success of a turnaround[5]
2. Bibeault's five stages for planning and conducting a turnaround[6]
3. Sloma's 13-step flowchart model to help organize and prioritize the turnaround process steps[7]
4. Goldstick's business health index, as modified for use in hospitals, to determine objectively the level of adversity[8]
5. Goldstick's system for classifying the corporation according to how well its strategy fits its environment[9]

6. Sloma's (a) catalog of key symptoms; (b) kit of macrotools; (c) kit of microtools; and (d) arsenal of remedial, restorative actions[10]

7. Strassmann's return on management ratio to determine the effectiveness of management[11]

8. Tomasko's zero based analysis of staff functions[12]

9. Tomasko's span of control analysis to identify excessive management[13]

10. Stewart's functional audit concept and his internal needs list approach[14]

In addition to these useful tools, the usual use is made of financial ratio analysis (especially trends), cash flow projections, and pro forma statements. Depending on need and the availability of information, a marketing audit might also be accomplished. Finally, key executives are evaluated using the tool illustrated in Exhibit 1.3 plus other personal judgments of their past and potential performance.

Turnaround Plan

When the initial evaluation has been completed, attention can be directed to the preparation of a comprehensive turnaround plan. This turnaround plan provides guidelines for the turnaround effort and is a base of measurable performance targets by which the turnaround effort can be measured. The quality and ultimate effectiveness of the organization's turnaround plan is directly related to the value and accuracy of the initial evaluation. If the diagnosis was sound, then the turnaround plan has a much greater chance of being successful.

The substance of a turnaround plan differs from situation to situation but the plan most commonly addresses

1. the prioritization of the major problems or issues identified during the evaluation phase;

2. turnaround objectives, strategies for achieving the objectives, and specific actions that must be taken;

3. parameters and standards for measuring turnaround success as well as benchmarks for evaluating turnaround progress;

4. contingency plans that address the most likely problem that might be encountered during the turnaround; and

5. provisions for beginning to position the organization for a return to growth.

The turnaround plan is survival focused. It is not a strategic plan, although strategic issues might be very much involved. When the plan is completed, it should be tested against the following criteria before it is implemented:

1. Is the plan focused on improving cash flow and restoring acceptable margins?
2. Does the plan reflect the best thinking of all concerned?
3. Are actions in the plan compatible with the aims, philosophy, and values of the stakeholders?
4. Is the plan simple, realistic, easily communicated, challenging, and doable?
5. Can the plan serve as a basis for measuring management's progress and thus serve as an incentive to stimulate motivation?

Implementing the Turnaround Plan

It is one thing to prepare a comprehensive turnaround plan but quite another to implement it successfully. Implementation will not likely go according to plan; however, the turnaround plan at least provides a basic structure from which necessary turnaround actions can be implemented. Things always go wrong, but without a plan, the process is likely to turn to chaos.

Before specific actions are taken to implement the turnaround plan, key linking processes must be put into place. Without these, the implementation of the plan runs a high risk of failure.

The Linking Processes

Throughout the turnaround implementation period, ultimate success depends a great deal on the effectiveness of three important linking processes: communication, problem solving, and decision making. These three processes are the organizational glue that binds the many diverse efforts taking place throughout the turnaround period. Each of these three crucial linking processes must be carefully planned, structured, and nurtured during the turnaround.

Communication. The usual channels and forms of communication that might be sufficient under ordinary circumstances are not effective in a turnaround. Extraordinary effort must be devoted to establishing effective communication channels. Likewise, special attention must be given to the forms of communication used. Finally, the messages communicated must be effective in getting attention, ensuring understanding, achieving commitment, and eliciting the desired supportive actions. The following forms of communication have proven most effective in turnaround:

1. *Meetings.* Meetings should be held throughout the process with all levels of stakeholders for the purposes of informing, persuading, or deciding. These include extensive meetings with employees.
2. *Written materials.* Designed for in-house use, these materials include candid personal letters to key individuals and to employees, information memorandums, special bulletins, special articles in the house organ, and other similar means of informing, persuading, and soliciting support for the turnaround effort.
3. *Information focal points.* Setting these up includes designating and staffing certain offices and certain specific locations (e.g., the entrance to the cafeteria and major employee work entrances and exits) as information centers.
4. *Hot lines.* Two forms of hot line are established. One is devoted to receiving questions, problems, or suggestions from anyone involved. The other is set aside for important messages from management and for prerecorded information to control rumors.
5. *Informal rounds.* Nothing is as effective as one-on-one, two-way communication. This communication is most effective if it is done at the employee's workplace; therefore, key executives and managers are assigned rounds throughout the facility on all work shifts.
6. *Public information.* Carefully prepared statements for public release as well as tailored communications to manage issues that arise are essential.

Problem solving. Problem-raising and problem-solving approaches cannot be left to chance during a turnaround. The informal methods previously used to solve problems have been disrupted by the turnaround effort and especially by the turnover of key individuals that usually occurs. It is therefore essential that all concerned know and agree to a process for raising problems and for resolving them when the turnaround is implemented.

The CEO and key executives will be consumed with major strategic and top-level operational problems; therefore, raising and resolving most problems should be delegated to the lowest level possible. This means clearly identifying which types of problems and under what circumstances problems are to be referred upward. Managers have a much greater tendency to delegate upward in a turnaround due to their own anxiety and insecurity. This tendency can be avoided by issuing problem-solving guidelines.

Decision making. Ad hoc decision teams, an administrative council, and a president's council can provide an effective deliberation and decision-making structure for problems that must be brought upward for resolution. The ad hoc teams function like a matrix organization. The administrative council, which consists of division executives, can facilitate most decisions by advising the chief operating officer (COO) or CEO. The president's council, which is comprised of the most senior executives, decides matters of major strategic and operational importance.

Role of the Turnaround Leader

As used in this chapter, a role is defined as a set of performance expectations of an individual executive holding a particular position in a specific organization at a given point in time. The role of the CEO in a turnaround or near turnaround can be summarized as follows:

1. To serve as the principal architect of the turnaround plan and to ensure its effective execution
2. To serve as a catalyst to constantly energize the turnaround process and to keep the turnaround momentum going
3. To provide overall leadership for and specific management of the turnaround process as it progresses through the usual stages
4. To create and maintain a supportive organizational climate for successful change and effective transition to the new organization to be created by the turnaround
5. To anticipate and plan for the support of affected employees by minimizing the impact of economic hardship and psychological trauma

In essence, the CEO must take the lead in providing leadership and in working effectively with all major stakeholders to generate support for the turnaround. To provide the impetus that will make the turnaround successful, all parties must fully empower the CEO to fulfill the role of turnaround leader and must totally support the CEO if he or she is to be successful in achieving a financially viable, socially responsive health care organization.

Nothing heals corporate wounds like success. The CEO should not feel guilty for using strong, often dictatorial, direction early in the turnaround process. Be ruthless in the pursuit of objectives, but be gracious with people.

Role of Other Key Stakeholders

Although the CEO has ultimate responsibility for the success (or lack of success) of the turnaround effort, it must be a team effort involving the board, the medical staff, other executives, directors, managers, employees, and volunteers. Support must also be garnered from unions, creditors, suppliers, contractors, third-party payers, and the community at large. All are of vital importance to the success of the turnaround, but space limitations prohibit describing the role of each. The turnaround leader would be wise to enlist their support and orchestrate their effort in helping to achieve a successful turnaround.

Specific Turnaround Actions

Actions that are taken in implementing the turnaround plan can be divided for discussion into two categories: urgent and sustaining. Urgent actions are those taken to improve the financial situation. Sustaining actions are those aimed at ensuring the long-term financial viability and future success of the organization.

Urgent actions. Urgent actions are those that are most likely to yield improved cash flow and operating margins. The first urgent action is usually to implement an operating adjustment plan, to include

1. the reduction or elimination of certain programs or services;
2. the consolidation of functions to reduce overhead;
3. general reductions in staffing;
4. reductions in contract costs through the elimination of the agreements or the reduction of the amounts;
5. the deferment of capital projects and purchases;

6. the reduction of material costs through prudent purchasing, the sale of excess inventory, and improved inventory management;
7. the reduction of perquisites and benefits;
8. the reduction of advertising and promotion expenses;
9. the elimination of overtime; and
10. other expense reductions where possible.

Two other urgent efforts include enhancing revenue and increasing cash flow. Actions might include price adjustments, the renegotiation of third-party contracts, the reevaluation of past cost reports to seek additional reimbursement, selling accounts receivable, refinancing long-term debt, and other such actions to improve overall financial performance. These actions are short term. They must be accompanied by more long-term sustaining efforts.

Sustaining actions. Bibeault refers to four sustaining elements that must be present if a turnaround is to be successful.[15] These include (1) new, competent top management with full authority to make required changes; (2) an economically and competitively viable core operation; (3) bridge capital from internal and external sources to provide financing during the turnaround period; and (4) motivated employees with a positive attitude. While these four core elements are as essential in a hospital turnaround as they are in a general business turnaround, they alone might not suffice in a hospital turnaround. In my judgment, there are ten core elements in a successful hospital turnaround. These core elements are

1. a new, fully supported statement of mission and organizational philosophy that provides clear meaning to the organization's purpose and serves as a blueprint for rebuilding the organization;
2. a definitive statement of a shared vision of the organization's desired future that provides a focal point for the talents and efforts of all those involved;
3. an overall business strategy that clearly pinpoints the distinctiveness of the organization, identifies its major service lines, stakes out the markets it seeks to capture, and provides an overall framework for the specific business plans of the organization;
4. an organizational structure that clearly delineates authority, responsibility, and individual accountability as well as providing

a process through which problems get identified, decisions get made in a timely manner, and desired results are achieved;

5. a skilled group of executives, directors, supervisors, and employees who work together as teams, who are dedicated to a successful turnaround, and who wish to grow with the organization as well as share in its successes;

6. a dedicated, effectively organized medical staff that shares and supports the goals of the turnaround effort and future vision of the organization;

7. a corporate culture that represents shared values that support the aims of the turnaround effort;

8. a physical plant and technology capable of supporting the medical staff and the patient care mission of the hospital;

9. a growing reserve of financial resources from which additional services can be developed and with which improvements in existing services can be made; and

10. a supportive community that shares the turnaround and postturnaround goals of the organization and lends its support in achieving these goals.

The pursuit of these ten core elements underlies the sustaining actions that the turnaround leader must take if the turnaround is to be successful in the long run.

External Factors

No organization operates in a vacuum. As a creation of the state, the corporation is publicly accountable. Since hospitals are social institutions, they have a special accountability. It then follows that in any hospital turnaround situation, factors and stakeholders external to the organization must be considered. These external considerations can be either positive or negative.

Creditors who will not cooperate, suppliers who will not give concessions, contractors who will not renegotiate, unions that pursue stonewalling as a strategy and third-party payers who press for deep discounts are among the many possible external factors that might negatively influence the outcome of a turnaround effort. Add to these the possibility of an aggressive business coalition, a noncooperative or even hostile news media, a less than supportive community, and aggressive competitors. Fortunately, this combination of negative factors is not commonplace. But, some of these factors are present in most turnaround situations, so the turnaround leader must be prepared to naturalize them.

Fortunately, in the turnarounds I have experienced, the external stakeholders have been largely supportive. Creditors were willing to accept some delays in payments. A number of contracts were favorably renegotiated. Unions were reasonable. Third-party contracts were settled as favorably as could be expected.

The turnarounds I experienced were also assisted by a supportive business community and by demanding but nonetheless supportive news media. Finally, the local and state political climates were supportive in that they presented no barriers.

External support cannot be taken for granted in a turnaround situation. The turnaround leader must usually take the lead in seeking this support. This means personal contact. Thorough staff work should be done before each meeting with a major external stakeholder. The objectives are to know each well, to project confidence, to present a plan that has credibility, and to gain the support needed for the organization's turnaround effort.

Remaining Challenges

When the management change, evaluation, emergency, and stabilization stages have been completed, the remaining challenge is to achieve what Bibeault refers to as the return-to-normal-growth stage.[16] This final stage is the most lengthy of the five stages. The challenges that remain are difficult, and they require a tremendous commitment of time and talent. In this final stage, efforts include

1. making the new mission, vision statements, and strategy operational;
2. completing a final restructuring of the corporation and redeployment of assets to future defined growth opportunities;
3. further developing a solid, supportive organizational culture;
4. building additional financial reserves for future expansion and improvements;
5. focusing major efforts on service responsiveness and quality;
6. ensuring further development of the organization's employees and giving greater attention to the quality of their work life; and

7. further developing the medical center-medical staff relationship as a partnership in serving the community's health care needs.

These sustaining, organizational renewal efforts will likely continue indefinitely.

Twenty-Twenty Hindsight

When turnarounds have been successful, there is usually little motivation to look back. It is human tendency to remember and celebrate our successes while repressing our mistakes. As a close to this chapter, two lists are presented. The first list highlights successes. The second addresses actions that did not meet expectations.

Successful Actions

This summary of turnaround actions that were successful does not imply that such actions are always successful. In fact, actions must always be tailored to the unique aspects of each situation. The most successful actions in my recent turnarounds were

1. the effective use of a structured transition process and transition task force to ensure quick integration of the new CEO into the organization;
2. the development and use of a conceptual framework modified from the literature for better understanding and planning of the turnaround process;
3. direct use of a number of diagnostic tools gleaned from the literature on corporate turnaround;
4. the development and use of a turnaround plan that guided actions and measured progress;
5. the establishment of communication, problem-solving, and decision-making processes before turnaround actions;
6. the pursuit of both urgent and sustaining actions simultaneously during the turnaround effort both to yield short-term gain and to establish a basis for future success.

Unsuccessful Actions

This second list of turnaround actions that were not as successful as expected does not represent actions that should never be taken because they might fail. Again, the particulars of each situation usually determine what succeeds and what fails. The least successful actions were

1. delaying and overextending the process of replacing key executives and directors who could not or would not contribute effectively to the success of the turnaround (the key is to quickly evaluate and replace those who must go);
2. delaying and overextending the operating adjustments process, especially in delaying announcements of employee layoffs (it should be done quickly, and all announcements should be made in one day; get employees out of the facility by handling outplacement at a remote site);
3. failing to follow up effectively on some major actions during the turnaround despite the fact that briefing books were established (due to the delays in replacing key people, at any given time, there just were not enough players on the field); and
4. spending too much time initially on process and debate rather than taking total control and making things happen more quickly (the key is to assume total empowerment, seize total control initially, and then become more participative in style when the emergency stage is completed).

Summary

Following a structured, systematic approach to planning and achieving a corporate turnaround by using models described in the literature as supplemental aids can bolster the experience of the turnaround leader. I found this somewhat more formal approach more effective in contrast to a more intuitive approach I used in a prior turnaround effort.

Notes

1. L. E. Greiner and R. O. Metzger, *Consulting to Management* (Englewood Cliffs, NJ: Prentice Hall, Inc., 1983), 230–47.
2. D. B. Bibeault, *Corporate Turnaround: How Managers Turn Losers into Winners* (New York: McGraw-Hill Book Company, 1982), 91–106.
3. R. S. Sloma, *The Turnaround Manager's Handbook* (New York: The Free Press, 1985), 2.
4. W. Bridges, "Managing Organizational Transitions," *Organizational Dynamics* 15, (Summer 1986): 24–33.

5. G. Goldstick, *Business Rx: How to Get in the Black and Stay There* (New York: John Wiley & Sons, 1988), 215.
6. Bibeault, *Corporate Turnaround,* 91–106.
7. Sloma, *Turnaround Handbook,* 2.
8. Goldstick, *Business Rx,* 11–19.
9. Ibid., 116.
10. Sloma, *Turnaround Handbook,* 205–12.
11. R. M. Tomasko, *Downsizing: Reshaping the Corporation for the Future* (New York: AMACOM, 1987), 62.
12. Ibid., 90–92.
13. Ibid., 169–73.
14. J. Stewart, Jr., *Managing a Successful Business Turnaround* (New York: AMACOM, 1984), 33–66.
15. Bibeault, *Corporate Turnaround,* 111–21.
16. Ibid., 106.

2

PUBLIC RELATIONS AND MARKETING ASPECTS OF A TURNAROUND

Richard D. Roodman and Cheryl Minckler

Editors' Note: Coauthored by the CEO and the director of public relations and marketing of the medical center described, this chapter offers insights on the public relations and marketing aspects of a turnaround. The breadth and depth of the marketing programs described make the chapter worthwhile reading for not only individuals in public relations and marketing but the health care executive who is attempting to work with the media and maximize the positive aspects of the organization to various external publics during a turnaround.

The Situation

Before the Turnaround

Valley Medical Center began as the Renton Hospital, built by the U.S. Government as a war emergency facility. The hospital opened in 1945 with 100 beds and 18 bassinets. In 1948, the hospital was purchased from the government and became the first public district hospital in the state of Washington and in the country. The name was subsequently changed to Valley General Hospital.

The hospital district population boomed during the war years, as did the number of practitioners at Valley General, some of whose credentials were not thoroughly investigated at the time. There was also a general opinion in the medical community that practitioners who were not quite good enough to succeed in Seattle settled for a practice at Valley. Despite the many positive aspects of the medical center, Valley General developed a negative reputation and an accompanying nickname, Death Valley. Although most of its physicians were actually good doctors, some more colorful ones became visible through their exploits. Thus the hospital nickname became more well known. Clearly, the hospital's poor image also affected its market share, as people chose alternative health care providers.

The hospital is located in Southeast King County, 12 miles from Seattle. The district incorporates both suburban and rural communities. The hospital serves an estimated population of 275,000, approximately 25 percent of the county.

In 1969, a new facility was opened with 254 beds. In 1982, headlines read "Cost to patients at VGH to rise an average 16%, VGH Commission Draws Flak Over Salary," and photos ran front page with community residents carrying signs reading "It's Cheaper to Die." Plans were announced to hire a new, young CEO from Oklahoma, at a competitive wage. Amidst a great deal of controversy over his age and his salary, Rich Roodman was hired as Valley Medical Center's administrator. Members of the community were doubtful, some even enraged. Hundreds of people came to the board meeting to protest his hiring, while the Seattle media broadcast the community's outrage. They simply did not like the hospital, or trust the board, and felt his salary would bankrupt the patients who had to use the facility. In the midst of lawsuits, bad press, a respected surgeon's untimely death with an operating room scrub technician in a local hotel, budget hikes, increasing charges, hundreds of letters to the editor, and still more bad press, the new CEO entered the Valley Medical Center arena. What was evident to all connected with the hospital became evident to the new CEO: things had to change; the changes made would be pivotal to the hospital's future if not its very survival.

Death Valley Days Are Over

Since 1983, the hospital has triumphed over its past reputation, due to a strong commitment to quality care and the communication of that commitment to the hospital community. As health care entered a new era of consumerism and competitiveness, Valley's board of commissioners and administration realized that the only way to survive—and even thrive—was to provide the highest quality care and to convey the hospital's commitment to quality to the health care consumer.

Table 2.1   Statistics from Valley Medical Center Before and After Turnaround

	1983	*1989*
Total patient days	62,077	72,179
Emergency visits	32,080	50,388
Outpatient visits	36,124	57,528
Live births	1,947	3,004
Outpatient surgeries	3,060	7,955

Valley has been attracting additional patient volumes to enable the price of the product, patient care, to become even more competitive by costing less. Additional volumes increase the hospital's ability to maintain quality and high patient care staffing ratios and provide the financial resources to acquire new equipment and facilities and to pay competitive wages. Between 1983 and 1989, Valley's market share increased from 549 to 998 admissions for every 1,000 total admissions to the three other hospitals in the area. In 1991, that figure increased to 1,059 admissions for every 1,000 admissions for the other three hospitals. The bottom line: Valley's aggressive marketing has enhanced its image and thus strengthened its share of patients coming to Valley Medical Center. Table 2.1 presents some statistical data to reinforce the effectiveness of marketing.

True commitment to quality has reaped great rewards for Valley Medical Center. The Joint Commission on Accreditation of Healthcare Organizations (JCAHO) reaccredited Valley for three years, and the Death Valley days are over. The hospital's overall image—the consumer's perspective of quality—has vastly improved. The 1989 survey of community residents (see Exhibit 2.1) demonstrates increasingly high regard for the hospital and medical staff.

The community now ranks Valley's quality of care above that of the competition. This opinion is believed to be a direct result of the hospital's recent investments in staff, programs, technology, and facilities—investments in quality.

Valley has earned the support of the community leadership in recent years. The hospital and the administrator have the backing of the local and civic leaders and generally strong editorial support from community newspapers. This is considerably noteworthy considering the cloud under which Roodman came to the community.

Exhibit 2.1   Excerpts from the 1989 Community Opinion Survey on
                    Reputation and Quality

Overall Reputation

Eighty-seven percent of those with an opinion described the
reputation of Valley Medical Center to be above average (absolutely
outstanding, excellent, or good), with an average rating of 4.4
(good). The residents of Kent gave the highest ratings (an average
of 4.6). Those who did not have an opinion were left out of the
tabulation.

Quality of Doctors

Eighty-nine percent of the respondents rated the doctors who practice
at Valley Medical Center as better than or as good as the doctors in
downtown Seattle. Ninety-four percent believe that Valley Medical
Center doctors are as good as or better than doctors at other South
King County hospitals. These proportions were consistent across all
areas surveyed.

How It Happened

The difference between effective and ineffective strategic planning is
characterized by (1) community involvement in that it is their plan, (2)
timely updates from sources ranging from forums to direct mail, and (3)
actually accomplishing the objectives. At Valley Medical Center, every
new employee is acquainted with the marketing program during orientation. Every department manager knows that marketing is significant and
that his or her performance as a head nurse, for example, is based in part
on the ability to market this area of responsibility to the hospital's
customer. The hospital volunteer group, hospital chaplains, the board of
trustees, and anyone who comes in contact with the hospital recognizes that
marketing the hospital's resources is a vital function of the hospital's long-
range strategic plan.

A comprehensive approach to marketing was started. Internal
marketing strategies directed at human resources were put into effect.
Employees were made members of the marketing sales force through the
initiation of the FACTS program. A FACTS pamphlet about the hospital's
history, philosophy, marketing, programs and services was written. Each
year the pamphlet is updated, and Valley's employees can take the 150-

question FACTS quiz and earn a dinner for two at a favorite restaurant. The result is an informed internal sales force that can answer questions, communicate specific messages, and cross-sell services. These people feel good about their hospital and can accurately share information with their families and friends.

The comprehensive marketing program was expected to improve the institution's image, inform various constituencies of programs and services the hospital offered, increase market share, provide additional financial resources, and enhance the overall price competitiveness of the medical center. With these expectations in mind, specific marketing strategies aimed at consumers were initiated.

Implementation of the Marketing Program

Short-Term Solution: Maximize Communication

The short-term survival strategy used at Valley was to maximize communication by gathering information, setting the direction, and communicating specific strategies both internally and externally. Of immediate importance to hospital leadership in early 1983 was to find out where they were. Direct mail pieces were sent to the hospital district residents and employees inviting anyone who had a complaint or concern about their hospital to come and have coffee with the new CEO. The administrator spent time listening to nearly 700 people over a few months' time. These coffee meetings became one of the primary information gathering tools on which changes were based. They were also the first step in community outreach—the community felt as if the hospital really did care; their comments did not fall on deaf ears. Letters and postcards continued to be sent to the community, employees, and the medical staff inviting input and challenging everyone to get involved in change. Participation was encouraged at all levels.

As more and more voices were heard, it became clear that change was necessary. The hospital's image reflected the culmination of years of bad feelings both internally and in the community. Results of the information gathering within the hospital community showed the absence of pride and the presence of indecision, lethargy, demoralization, and insecurity. The administration knew from discussions that it must change the climate and the corporate culture and reinstate pride, interest, value, and excitement by fostering innovation: to somehow change the old way of doing things. A long-range tool was developed to get people involved.

Long-Term Survival Strategy: Marketing Community Affairs

The direction the administration chose to take was two-fold: (1) strategic long-range planning using the gathered information to set the direction with structure and organization and (2) the implementation of marketing to meet strategic long range goals.

While marketing had a highly visible external role through advertising, community programs, public affairs, public relations, and so on, it also needed to play an equally big role inside the hospital through customer relations, employee orientation, in-service education, and internal publications. Marketing encompasses consumer research, planning and development, and market positioning, along with publications, graphics, and design.

While there may be one focal point for marketing and related public relations functions, the successful marketing program had to become a key ingredient within each area, department, wing, or unit throughout the hospital. Each of the hospital's managers was asked to have a specific marketing goal for their department. Throughout the hospital, successful managers were rewarded for their involvement in the marketing function and their accomplishment of specific goals. The administration found it desirable to identify marketing as one of the five cornerstones for hospital management. It became clear that there needed to be one area within the hospital organization that had the ultimate role for coordinating all the marketing functions throughout the hospital. For this department to be successful, it would need full support from the administration, visibility throughout the medical center, and the participation of all departments. The public relations department added a marketing element, under the direction of the assistant administrator of community affairs and marketing.

Comprehensive Approach: Internal and External Marketing

Internally, management focused first on the existing corporate structure and began striving to innovate wherever possible. A strategic long-range planning process was used to set the direction and provide some structure in the organization.

In 1983, the administration implemented an ambitious long-range strategic planning process. The eight-month process involved over 500 people: employees at all levels, physicians, citizens and business leaders of the community, volunteers, the auxiliary, and elected officials. They collectively grappled with issues including the health care needs of the community, the mission and role of the hospital, how to set and maintain standards for quality control, and their vision of the hospital's future role in the community.

The result of their efforts was a five-year long-range strategic plan. Since 1984, this document has been reviewed each year and has served as the basis for the hospital's annual goals and objectives. The plan was distributed to everyone associated with the hospital. The extensive employee and community involvement in the planning process proved so successful that in October 1988, another five-year long-range strategic plan was produced following a similar procedure.

Valley's mission statement resulted from the planning process of 1983. It prioritizes and formally acknowledges the hospital's dedication to quality patient care. Quality patient care at Valley is demonstrated through high staff-patient ratios; state-of-the-art technology; joint ventures with other hospitals; and excellent medical staff, facilities, and programs. The hospital is also dedicated to clear and consistent communications with all constituencies: medical staff, employees, volunteers, physicians and their office staff, and the community.

Streamlining the Administrative Staff

The executive administrative staff in any hospital usually consists of the COO, director of nursing, chief financial officer (CFO), perhaps a director of technical services, perhaps a director of support services, a medical director, a director of community affairs, a director of marketing, and a director of human resources. Before the hospital plunged into a visible marketing philosophy, three top management positions were reduced. It was helpful to eliminate or reduce these positions before spending a lot of money on marketing; it made it easier for employees, medical staff, and the community in general to swallow new programs such as marketing when the administrative staff was small.

Shaping the Management Team

Once the administrative staff was streamlined and educated about marketing, it became necessary to bring along the rest of the hospital by incorporating additional management personnel into the effort. Department heads and supervisors were made accountable for a variety of variables to remain employed and be candidates for a raise. Their annual evaluation is based on their ability to accomplish goals and objectives within each one of these areas. Since department heads can either make or break a hospital, a supportive management team, like the one at Valley, is a tremendous resource.

Funding

Seven months into each year of the budget cycle the CEO, CFO, and the community affairs and marketing representatives meet. Over several meetings, the marketing objectives of the next year are planned. At that time, a determination is made to either maintain or increase the marketing budget for the coming year.

Evaluation of Marketing

We have several ways of evaluating the success of our marketing efforts: patient activity (admissions, emergency room visits, obstetrics, inpatient and outpatient surgeries, outpatient visits, etc.); public opinion surveys conducted every 18 months; patient representative surveys of inpatients and outpatients; and the use of the physician referral line (which increased from 150 calls per month in 1983 to 900 calls per month in 1989).

The hospital, under the administration's care, has enjoyed six years of phenomenal growth in an era plagued with uncertainty. The hospital has been able to attract an increasing number of full-paying patients through its award-winning marketing efforts, especially in consumer-driven areas such as obstetrics and emergency services. Both of these areas have grown over 50 percent since Roodman's arrival. Valley now delivers 3,000 babies each year and experiences 50,000 emergency room visits per year. Valley's outpatient surgical procedures have grown from 250 per month to 700 per month. As a result of increases in volume, the impact on the hospital's rates due to contractual allowances has been minimized. The Washington State Rate Commission has referenced Valley as a low cost provider as a result of its increases in market share generated by consumer support, preferred provider status and cost-effective management. Additionally, this increase in market share has lead to increased profits for the hospital, despite Valley's location in a rate-regulated state. The hospital doubled its profits in two years and has continued to project major increases.

Internal Elements of the Marketing Plan

Management by Walking Around

The CEO has been actively involved in the development and implementation of activities in most successful functions in the hospital. As this philosophy relates to marketing, it's critical that the CEO do more than merely support the marketing function. For the marketing activities to have a chance at success, the CEO must be actively involved.

Quite a bit has been written lately about management by walking around. A successful marketing program stands a better chance of success when the administrator visibly gets around the facility and has exchanges with all the various constituents connected with the hospital. Through this personal interaction, the administrator can respond to questions about the marketing program and reinforce and validate various campaign and marketing strategies the hospital is trying to implement. It is also helpful to the marketing program and the administration if the administrator keeps both ears and eyes open and gets to know a variety of people inside and outside the hospital. This approach has been tremendous in allowing Valley's administrator to obtain first-hand information about things that employees, patients, and doctors feel are important.

Communication of the Marketing Plan to the Internal Community

One technique for breaking down the politics of marketing and avoiding the ramifications of people being surprised is to develop displays regarding various campaigns before they actually become visible in the community. It has been helpful to get an actual busboard poster (an advertisement on the side or back of a bus) and display it in the lobby a couple of weeks before the campaign actually begins to run. If the campaign employs other marketing elements such as billboards, print ads, and television or radio announcements as well as busboards, the public relations department creates a mixed media display, which is placed at several key locations within the hospital. No one is taken by surprise. An informed work force can become a supportive element in any hospital's overall marketing campaign.

Involvement of Human Resources

Once the hospital had established what it stood for, it became critical to gain acceptance and understanding from the medical staff, the employees, the managers, the board of trustees, and all who are related to the hospital. One way of accomplishing this objective is to publish a document that outlines exactly what the administration and planning group feels the hospital stands for along with a variety of other features about the hospital. It is produced in a format that is available to various groups within the hospital. At Valley Medical Center, the administration gained a high level of understanding, acceptance, and support by developing and publishing what everyone now knows as the FACTS pamphlet. The first FACTS pamphlet described programs, services, the hospital's mission and role, a positioning statement, and other important information about Valley Medical Center. It has grown into a 44-page booklet, updated and published annually, containing information on everything about the hospital relevant to its past, present, and future. The FACTS pamphlet is offered to all employees, physicians and medical support staff, volunteers, and chaplains as a means to learn more about the hospital.

After developing the FACTS pamphlet, this marketing opportunity was taken a step further, by asking the finer restaurants in the Seattle areas if they would be willing to participate by donating a $50 dinner-for-two certificate for every two or three dinners the hospital purchased. The restaurants liked the idea, so Valley offered the certificates as prizes for members of various hospital groups who took the time to read the FACTS pamphlet and take the FACTS quiz. The results of this annual program have been outstanding and unprecedented. Each year, over 2,000 people are exposed to why Valley Medical Center is a wonderful place to work, refer patients, and volunteer time. These same people understand Valley's positioning statement and services. Employees have the opportunity and incentive to learn more about their hospital and, in turn, to promote those facts to our customers.

External Elements of the Marketing Plan

Facilities Development

In 1984, a $23 million expansion program was completed, bringing the licensed bed capacity to 303. The name was changed to Valley Medical Center to better reflect the comprehensive services offered. Our hospital continues to receive many compliments from patients and guests, including professional designers and architects. Over the past few years, landscaping and the addition of new colors and furnishings have improved the overall appearance of the medical center.

Campus development and expansion includes the 100,000-square foot-Talbot Professional Center. This medical office building is owned and developed by a partnership of our staff physicians. They lease the building site from Valley Medical Center which in turn sublease the first floor of the office building for the fitness center.

Community Education

To improve the quality of life in the community, the hospital offers a variety of classes and health events, ranging from cardiopulmonary resuscitation and weight loss programs to a Healthy Baby Week filled with activities. Many of these programs are offered free of charge.

Community Service

In 1986, when most hospitals were cutting back on teaching programs, Valley began a Family Practice Residency program to meet the growing need for maternity and indigent care and to increase the hospital's quality of care through the program's educational emphasis. The hospital's commitment to quality extends to the indigent in the community. The Valley Share Program (a cooperative venture of the County Health Department, Valley, and its staff physicians) refers low-income women to the hospital for delivery and postnatal care, which Valley provides on an ability-to-pay basis. In 1987, there were 207 deliveries at Valley through the Family Practice Residency Program. Ninety-two percent of the deliveries were indigent cases.

Marketing Strategies Aimed at Individual Consumers

Baby Pager. Valley was looking for a way to further promote its Birth Center, one of a number of Centers of Excellence within the hospital. The challenge was to come up with an innovative promotional campaign to attract the attention of parents-to-be. A common concern is, Where and how will I contact my spouse when it's time? Valley decided to offer Baby Pagers to expectant parents and to advertise the pager with a television commercial. The commercial is a take-off on the 1939 film starring Jeanette McDonald and Nelson Eddy in their family "love call." Since November 1987, Valley has been offering the free use of a pager to couples in the final two months of pregnancy with a fully refundable $40 deposit. The pagers have been extremely popular, and hundreds are loaned to expectant couples each year. The pagers are a fond memory for many parents, and their paging stories keep coming in.

Rapid Care. Approximately 80 percent of Valley's emergency department visits are not emergencies. The most frequent complaints involve delays in diagnosis and treatment. To solve the problem, Valley instituted Rapid

Care, a care delivery program for patients with problems that can be adequately evaluated and treated in less than 60 minutes. Patients are evaluated by the triage nurse. He or she determines if the chief complaint meets Rapid Care criteria. Rapid Care, begun in August 1987, is housed within the emergency department and staffed by one doctor, one nurse and one medical-surgical technician. Rapid Care allows the emergency department to function more effectively by freeing up emergency treatment rooms and staff for more critical situations, better enabling them to meet the demands of an increasing patient population. Time slips indicate the program is working: Rapid Care patients average 59 to 69 minutes per visit from the time they walk in the door to the time they exit. Emergency visits increased an impressive 43 percent from 1985.

Goldencare at Valley. Begun in September 1986, Goldencare at Valley is a free program for adults aged 65 and older who carry Medicare Parts A and B with approved supplemental insurance. The program guarantees that members will never receive a hospital bill; the program absorbs the remaining charges not paid by Medicare or the supplemental insurance. In addition, members receive free reserved parking, one-on-one assistance with medical paperwork, discounts at various service and retail outlets; and free senior workshops. The program had 6,000 members at the end of 1989 and is experiencing a growth rate of approximately 100 new members a month. Approximately 50 percent have been admitted as patients. It is seen as a valuable community service program and public relations tool.

Visits to new mothers. This program is affectionately known around the hospital as Roses from Rich. Administrator Rich Roodman personally visits each new mother, asks about her care at Valley, and presents her with a long-stemmed rose and congratulatory card. While this program has no direct impact on the bottom line, the gesture helps increase Valley's image as a caring institution and gives valuable, immediate feedback on the quality of obstetric care.

Direct Mail

At Valley, direct mail is used quite extensively and is the most effective means for taking a message to a particular type of consumer because it is possible to demographically segment the target audience. In other words, direct mail offers greater control over who is exposed to the message than print, outdoor, or electronic media. The only routine exception to demographically segmenting the audience by age is Valley's bimonthly newsletter, *The Report to the Community.* This piece is mailed to approximately 175,000 community residences in the service area, people referred to as closest friends. This piece is direct mailed so extensively because each issue describes a specific center of medical excellence to the entire consumer audience that either does or might use Valley's services. Since the message in each newsletter issue only hits the consumer once, Valley depends on the frequency and regularity of *The Report's* mailing to build a positive image for the hospital. Since consumers only read about each center of medical excellence once, they probably do not remember all the details about each center, but more importantly, they might remember that Valley Medical Center has state-of-the-art Centers of Medical Excellence, which is often the most important image to establish.

Distribution of Community Newsletter and Physician Directory

In 1986, a new door-to-door delivery program was developed for *The Report* and the *Physician Directory.* The program serves as a fund-raiser for local youth groups (i.e., they are paid to deliver it) and saves the hospital approximately 50 percent over the cost of mailing these materials. It has the added advantage of reaching new and more mobile residents (e.g., apartment dwellers) and gives people the opportunity to ask questions of Valley's young ambassadors. (Before the students go out to deliver, they are educated about the hospital as part of the program.) In 1983, 23,000 copies of each issue of *The Report* (to apartments only; it was mailed to homes) and 150,000 copies of the *Physician Directory* were delivered door to door. A consumer research survey, conducted in the third quarter of 1987, indicated *The Report* was read and retained by three out of five residents; one in three retained a copy of the *Physician Directory.* The door-to-door program has been instrumental in the hospital's tremendous growth in market share for elective services.

MED-INFO

MED-INFO is a medical information telephone service that was developed as a joint venture between Valley hospital and a noncompeting hospital to the north of metropolitan Seattle during 1986. The call-in service provides an additional means for consumers to obtain referrals to all the hospitals' services, programs, educational classes, and support groups. This type of a program is a real community service and another mechanism for the consumer to access Valley's health care system

The Health Center Kiosk

Valley recently had a kiosk built and placed in a local shopping mall to serve as a community outreach health center. The kiosk is a means of promoting the hospital and physicians on staff. Services include cholesterol, blood pressure, blood sugar, and lung testing; nutrition information and analysis; and physician referral. Free health information and physician directories are distributed. There is a minimal charge for cholesterol screening; all other services are provided free of charge. The kiosk is staffed by an experienced hospital nurse and physician referral coordinator for one and two week periods throughout the year. In the first six weeks, more than 2,500 people visited the health center, and $9,000 was generated through cholesterol screening, enabling the kiosk to pay for itself.

Marketing Strategies Related to the Medical Staff

The **Physician Directory.** The *Physician Directory* is an annual publication in a booklet format with active and associate medical staff physicians' photographs as well as their names, addresses, and phone numbers. It is organized by specialty and subspecialty and has an alphabetical listing in back. The directory also contains other information about the medical staff, tells the reader how to get a referral to a Valley Medical Center doctor, and gives important phone numbers for the hospital's major departments. While the directory was designed primarily for use by the general public, it also serves as a reference guide for use by all hospital volunteers, employees, and medical staff offices. Thus, what began as a simple listing of physicians has grown into an information guide about the medical center as well.

The free physician referral service. The free physician referral service links new residents in the area to members of Valley's medical staff. Presently, about 800 calls are received a month from people looking for a physician for themselves or their families. The service offers names of physicians based on the desired office location, specialty requested, and any special needs.

The speakers bureau. Many hospitals now have speakers bureaus to help promote their medical staffs and to address a community need for this type of service. Valley has found it to be an active community resource through which speakers address local businesses and civic groups on a wide variety of medical and health topics. These topics can range from rheumatism to cataract surgery to stress management.

The speakers bureau is designed to incorporate both our medical staff and our professional services staff, providing an effective means for doctors to directly market themselves to specific groups and for employees at Valley to promote the hospital. In putting together the speakers bureau, nearly 100 percent of Valley's medical staff responded that they were interested in participating in the program. It continues to be a way for the physicians to have a high degree of visibility in the community and a means to market their specific specialties and interests.

Joint ventures. Many of the leading medical centers in the United States have been entering into joint ventures with their medical staffs for a number of years, as has Valley Medical Center. The purpose is to obtain mutual financial benefits and at the same time enhance the services to the community. For a joint venture to be successful, there must be (1) mutual trust and respect, (2) financial incentives, and (3) benefit to the community. Not all joint ventures are viable, and probably nine out of ten potential ideas will never be jointly developed.

A number of joint ventures came into being once Valley's long-range strategic plan was in place: outpatient x-ray services in which the physicians bought the equipment and the hospital provided the building; First Choice physician provider organization in which the physicians on staff along with doctors at six other hospitals combined with the participating hospitals to contribute capital to form a wholly-owned alternative delivery system; a medical office building on Valley's campus developed as a partnership in which members of Valley's active staff can take an equity position (i.e., buy space in the building) and the hospital leases the land; and the joint acquisition of laser equipment with Valley's ophthalmologists. A satellite clinic provides quality family and minor injury care to residents in the north end of the primary service area.

Groups Called into Action

Role of the Board

At Valley the board has been most supportive of marketing and its function within the medical center community. It is absolutely critical that the board of trustees of the hospital understand the marketing function and that they have some sensitivity to what the marketing department and the administration of the hospital expects to do in the marketing field during any period of time. Trustees are typically people from the community who must be in a position to speak up and defend the hospital's position as they circulate throughout the community. Since marketing is a relatively new field, it becomes even more important for board members to understand not only why hospitals must market but also the impact that a successful marketing campaign can have on the hospital and in turn the community. Once the board members understand that greater patient volumes generated through marketing can, in turn, mean lower unit costs and thus lower charges, they typically come around and can be a hospital administrator's greatest advocates when it comes to marketing. At Valley, the board participates in the marketing program by authoring regular reports in the bimonthly newsletter to the community. Additionally, two of the five trustees have actually been on billboards, busboards, newspapers, radio, and television.

Role of the Top Management Team

In addition to the 1982 streamlining of administrative and managerial staff, the administrator implemented a program to increase performance. In 1985 employees at all levels were asked to increase productivity by five percent. Employees were asked to think of ways to improve performance and productivity and to submit their ideas to their supervisor within five days. They were then given five months to increase productivity. The results were tremendous; Valley calculates that it saved $1.9 million annually through the implementation of this program.

Role of the Medical Staff

Physicians play an important role in the success of any hospital. Therefore, in the course of selling the hospital and its services, facilities, and overall program to all of the constituents, particular attention and focus should always be given to the medical staff. It is of primary importance to continually communicate with the medical staff, keeping them informed and including them in decision making whenever possible. The administration communicates with the physicians in a number of ways: one-on-one visits in the doctors' lounges; chatting with them in the hallways and the hospital's restaurant; sending letters directly to their homes or memos to their offices; eliciting their participation in the FACTS program; and basically trying to facilitate clear communication as much as possible. Since physicians are the quarterbacks who make the calls that govern (to some degree) what a hospital will and will not—or can and cannot—do, it is imperative that they buy in to marketing and that, in turn, the administration communicates to them what the hospital can do for loyal, supportive physicians.

The Role of Employees

The FACTS pamphlet ideas were among the first to emerge in the information gathering of 1983. Administration quickly put the idea into action, to initiate internal marketing right way. With over 1,500 employees at the hospital, it is important to keep them informed on what administration is doing and why. Employees can have a tremendous impact when they all pull together. The administration of the hospital and the marketing department take every opportunity to communicate the need for marketing and various promotional campaigns to the hospital's constituency. Supportive leaders—department heads, administrative staff, and board members—are helpful to the hospital's marketing program. At Valley, the employees are kept informed through letters mailed directly to their homes. Any good marketing effort stands to benefit if the marketing department and administration get the hospital work force to support it.

Role of Volunteers

Valley has found it advantageous to keep the volunteers up to speed with everything that is going on in the hospital. They are on the mailing list and receive newspaper clippings about the hospital, and the administration tries to speak with them every time it gets a chance. Most volunteer groups have steering committees, operating committees, or boards. It's a good idea to keep these people additionally informed and to win their endorsement when it comes time for volunteer groups to back a particular project at the hospital or to join the hospital's marketing plan.

Volunteers are frequently involved in services throughout the hospital where they have patient, employee, and visitor contact; they also present the opportunity to spread the good reputation throughout the community. It is therefore extremely important for them to understand the key marketing ideas, the advantages of your institution over competing institutions, and the process for selecting a physician from the physician referral service.

At Valley, the volunteers are incorporated into the greeter service. They wear special coats and red corsages, greeting people at the main entrance. The volunteers help incoming patients and families with information, show them to the admitting office, and even help patients in wheelchairs to the nursing units.

The umbrella organization that encompasses all facets of volunteer activity at Valley is called Volunteers in Action (VIA). This organization includes volunteers involved in special-events fund-raising, those who operate and oversee the gift shop, and all in-service volunteers, including junior volunteers. In addition to the greeter service, in-service volunteers staff the surgery and main information desks, provide an extra touch of caring on nursing units, and staff the courtesy cart that picks up arriving patients and visitors in the parking lot and takes them to the front door. They extend both the care and convenience of Valley to guests as soon as they arrive in the parking lot.

Role of the Consumers Advisory Council

The council is a sounding board and provides feedback from the community to the elected board of commissioners. The feedback is a form of education and a two-way communication function. Before the hospital implements significant new services, it periodically brings together the council members to review and discuss the projects. The administration also provides the Consumers Advisory Council with a list of goals and objectives each year to keep them informed and to get their feedback. Valley employees and volunteers can submit names of positive, forward-thinking, and knowledgeable people to participate on the council. Most recently, the Consumers Advisory Council has been an active participant in long-range planning for the hospital.

Role of the Press and Public Relations

At Valley, marketing established a foundation of positive feelings within the hospital community, while media and public relations managed the positive image. After the new CEO reestablished the organizational identity, the press followed up with close coverage of Valley's turnaround. The media's actions worked in Valley's favor by persuading the audience that the medical center was working to better the quality of care provided to the community. The wide acceptance of Valley Medical Center as the area's most comprehensive, convenient, quality health care provider close to home is due then, in part, to the work of the media.

Role of Other Hospitals

While competition has increased in the health care industry, networking with other area hospitals has brought Valley many positive opportunities.

Joint ventures with nearby hospitals have provided community residents with the highest quality care available in the area, both in pediatrics and oncology. By bringing the leaders in the fields onto Valley's campus, competition with those leading hospitals is diminished, volume is increased, and Valley can be extremely competitive with other area hospitals. Additionally, Valley has improved its image and, in turn, its market share, by associating with these other brand-name institutions.

Other Key Factors in the Turnaround

The employees, managers, medical staff, and board of directors' confidence and support of both administration and marketing has propelled Valley Medical Center into a leading role in the industry. By allowing the administrator to take risks and meet hurdles, the original vision has become a reality.

Remaining Challenges in the Turnaround

Maintenance is the main step necessary to continue the administration's improvement achieved in the turnaround. Valley experienced phenomenal turnaround since 1983. Yet instead of sitting back and enjoying the results of innovation, administration pushes ahead each year with new programs like the Southcenter Mall kiosk and Roses from Rich.

In addition, continuing to meet the high expectations of the community and maintaining an open and fair relationship with the media is critical to Valley's maintenance of the hospital turnaround.

Hindsight

In retrospect, the best action the administrator took was to involve as many people as possible in the turnaround, both internally and externally. Innovations such as the FACTS program, joint ventures with hospital physicians, and participation in marketing at all levels pulled the employees, medical staff, volunteers, and board of directors together to move toward a common goal. The key points of Valley's turnaround: Start positive changes on the inside and work outwards; be innovative; keep the board visible; maintain an open and fair relationship with the news media. The result was that community residents gradually began to see and feel the positive actions being taken. As work spread, community participation in educational programs, community forums, the volunteer groups, and health-related promotional events grew. Because of the participation of the medical staff, employees, board of directors, managers, and even the community in Valley's turnaround, everyone has ownership and pride in the hospital's success. That pride in the institution will keep Valley's family pushing ahead to initiate changes—changes that will carry Valley Medical Center through the 1990s.

3

TURNAROUND STRATEGY IN A
HEALTH CARE SYSTEM

Alethea O. Caldwell

Editors' Note: This chapter is one of the most comprehensive in the book. It describes the overall strategy of a turnaround of a health care system and management's role in that turnaround. It also describes the role of the medical staff and the community's involvement. Particular attention is given to the financial strategy for improving the organization's financial performance. In addition, the reorganization and streamlining of management is described. The accountability process and its importance to the overall turnaround are also presented.

The Situation

Had it not been for an unparalleled commitment to its mission to serve the poor and disadvantaged and a sheer determination to survive, Ancilla Systems Incorporated (ASI) would surely have perished before embarking on its present course of restructuring and turnaround.

Whatever could go wrong did go wrong for this proud, 120-year-old Catholic health care system headquartered just outside Chicago in Elk Grove Village, Illinois. Plagued by a series of internal and external crises, not the least of which were the drastic changes and reductions in reimbursement within the industry, ASI struggled to keep its footing in a changing and turbulent environment for which it, like many others, was unprepared.

That is not to say there was nothing right about ASI. Its major strength at that time was its dedicated people who operated with good intentions and a strong sense of mission. That mission stemmed from ASI's origins and its sponsor, the Poor Handmaids of Jesus Christ, or Ancilla Domini Sisters, Inc. The history of the Poor Handmaids began in the village of Dernbach, Germany, in 1851 with Sister Mary Katherine Kasper, who began a little house to care for the poor and sick. She was joined by other young women, and their work spread to other countries. The Poor Handmaids came to the United States in 1869 and established their first mission in Ft. Wayne, Indiana. St. Joseph's Hospital there is the present physical evidence of their humble beginnings.

From Ft. Wayne they spread their mission to Chicago's West Side, where the system has recently closed its St. Anne's Hospital but still operates St. Elizabeth's Hospital.

Other religious groups that sponsor health care institutions have spread their missions to include broad socioeconomic groups into their bases of operation. The Poor Handmaids, however, have traditionally maintained a physical presence in areas of need and poverty. In addition to the Ft. Wayne, Indiana, and Chicago facilities already mentioned, ASI operates St. Mary's Hospital in East St. Louis, Illinois, currently recognized as one of the nation's most economically depressed areas; St. Mary Medical Center in Gary, and St. Catherine's Hospital, East Chicago, both of which are situated in northwest Indiana, a region that has never fully recovered from the ramifications of the nation's failing steel industry; and two Indiana facilities in less urban settings, St. Mary Medical Center, Hobart, and Saint Joseph Hospital, Mishawaka. The system also operates various other health care subsidiaries including a home health division.

From 1982 to 1986 a multitude of problems within the system led to several crises. These were caused by insufficient action and a lack of aggressive leadership in addressing the early symptoms and subsequent problems.

The immediate crises included bank notes for the Chicago affiliates coming due; significant cash, drains on the system created by losses of two now-closed Chicago hospitals, St. Anne's and its sister hospital, St. Anne's West; St. Elizabeth's inaccessibility to any substantial amount of the system's cash, which was tied up in receivables; the risk of acceleration of a portion of the Indiana group's long-term debt; and the reductions in reimbursement for indigent care programs that occurred with the adoption of the Medicaid contracting program in Illinois.

The system began to experience declines in profitability leading to losses in 1985 and 1986. Critical organizational divisions and tensions existed between the holding corporation and the hospital corporations. The system had lost the capability to provide adequate capital to the affiliates to enable them to acquire up-to-date technology and other amenities to keep them competitive within their markets. Costs within the system were high compared with other systems and facilities operating in the same areas.

A large portion of Ancilla's problems were due to the service locations and patient mix of the affiliates. About 66 percent of all patients served throughout the system in 1987 were beneficiaries of either Medicare or Medicaid. In 1988 that figure stood at about 60 percent. Slightly more than 30 percent of the system's revenue was derived from commercial insurers for the two-year period. A geographic overview shows ASI facilities to be in generally undesirable locations due to poor economic conditions of the areas served. Market positions for the affiliates were not strong. The various financial, management, data, and other systems supporting the hospitals were out of date. Standardization did not exist, making it impossible to compare and analyze the depth of the problems. Thus, affiliate hospital leadership did not have the resources or capital to correct the problems rapidly enough. As was the case at the system level, aggressive, timely action was often absent among the affiliates.

While this network of hospitals technically formed a system, Ancilla had many of the disadvantages of system organization but not enough advantages to make it a viable player in the changing health care environment. ASI had not truly been integrated into a system.

The system was restructured in 1984, with an attempt to consolidate its governance and management. Regional strategies and solutions were introduced but never implemented effectively. The concept of Catholic hospitals seeking shared solutions to maintain viability was introduced within the Chicago service area, but no substantial collaborative partnerships emerged. Some improvements did occur, but there were still eight separate corporations with various governing combinations. The results were continuing conflicts concerning authority and responsibility due to the complex corporate structure and continued high system costs with barriers to the flow of funds. In 1984 the system also adopted a strategic plan that called for a reduction of its acute care presence in the competitive Chicago market and a strengthening of the system presence in its other markets through service reconfiguration and collaborative alignments. That plan was never implemented.

Between the 1984 restructuring and the recognition of impending crisis in 1987, Ancilla's affiliates, along with the industry as a whole, experienced drastic revisions in reimbursement and methodology, severe reductions in utilization, and increases in the scope and form of competition.

Despite some success in creating financial interdependence, the system formed in 1984 did not meet its financial or strategic planning goals. There were intensive capital formation efforts, but overall financial strength continued to seriously deteriorate. Management perspectives were narrow, in-depth financial management was lacking, and there was critical need for a reevaluation of the system's product lines and the roles of the individual hospitals within their respective communities.

System governance recognized the critical condition and the need to seek leadership that could gather the mix of skills and expertise needed to assess the system, determine its long term viability, prioritize its problems, and develop a plan of attack. To that end, a national leadership search was conducted. The sponsor specifically sought an individual with expertise in turnaround skills who also possessed the ability to identify viable elements within the system. The mandate of the president and CEO would be to resolve the Chicago hospital crisis, renegotiate the debt on both St. Anne's and St. Anne's West, complete the divestiture of St. Anne's West, stabilize the remaining system hospitals, and, if possible, develop or modify strategic alternatives for the survival of the system and its mission in some form. Almost immediately following the selection of the new president and CEO of Ancilla Systems, the first steps were taken toward the restructuring of a new organization that could begin to deal with its problems.

The Approach

There were strategic, operational, and financial elements to ASI's turnaround, making its scope more difficult to gauge. The first action taken was a complete assessment of the organization, which included an evaluation of

- the external environment—economic, social, and governmental;
- financial performance indicators;
- medical staff strengths and weaknesses;
- governance, ownership, and management structures;
- service and program configuration;
- human resource strengths and weaknesses;
- overall quality review and control;
- cash management;
- asset deployment;
- capacity issues;

- reimbursement and pricing strategies;
- revenue generating opportunities;
- cost-reduction approaches;
- customer satisfaction;
- risk management for business and liability insurance needs;
- financing capability and debt structure; and
- information system and decision support effectiveness.

The assessment phase also involved an analysis of the system's governance structure, which included a review of the mission and purpose of the organization; an analysis of strategic directives; and an examination of executive management. A comprehensive and multifaceted systemwide survey project was also undertaken to analyze existing community perceptions, patient satisfaction levels, employee opinions, and medical staff opinions and perceptions.

The findings of the overall assessment resulted in (1) the corporate restructuring into four regional boards with accountability to a single ASI board, (2) a downsized organization that included the corporate office and all the affiliates, and (3) the divestiture of St. Anne's West and the closure of St. Anne's.

Restructuring

Restructuring to a regional approach streamlined governance and decision making and facilitated the transfer of affiliate assets within each region. Equivalent divisions at each affiliate were created to maintain local focus on issues such as quality assurance and community development programs that would meet local needs. In addition, the bylaws were restructured to clarify and strengthen the reserved powers of the holding company and sponsor to make more precise the relationships of governance and management at the system and affiliate level and strengthen the ability of the system to respond to opportunities and challenges. To this end, revisions such as the inclusion of the wording ". . . and support the other entities within the health system. . . ." were added to the objective and purpose section of each region's corporate bylaws document. Other changes involved the expansion of ASI's authority or the addition of approval powers that had already been granted. The new approvals and establishment of more clearly enunciated policies and procedures were intended to reduce some of the existing friction between affiliate and

Figure 3.1   Regional Structure

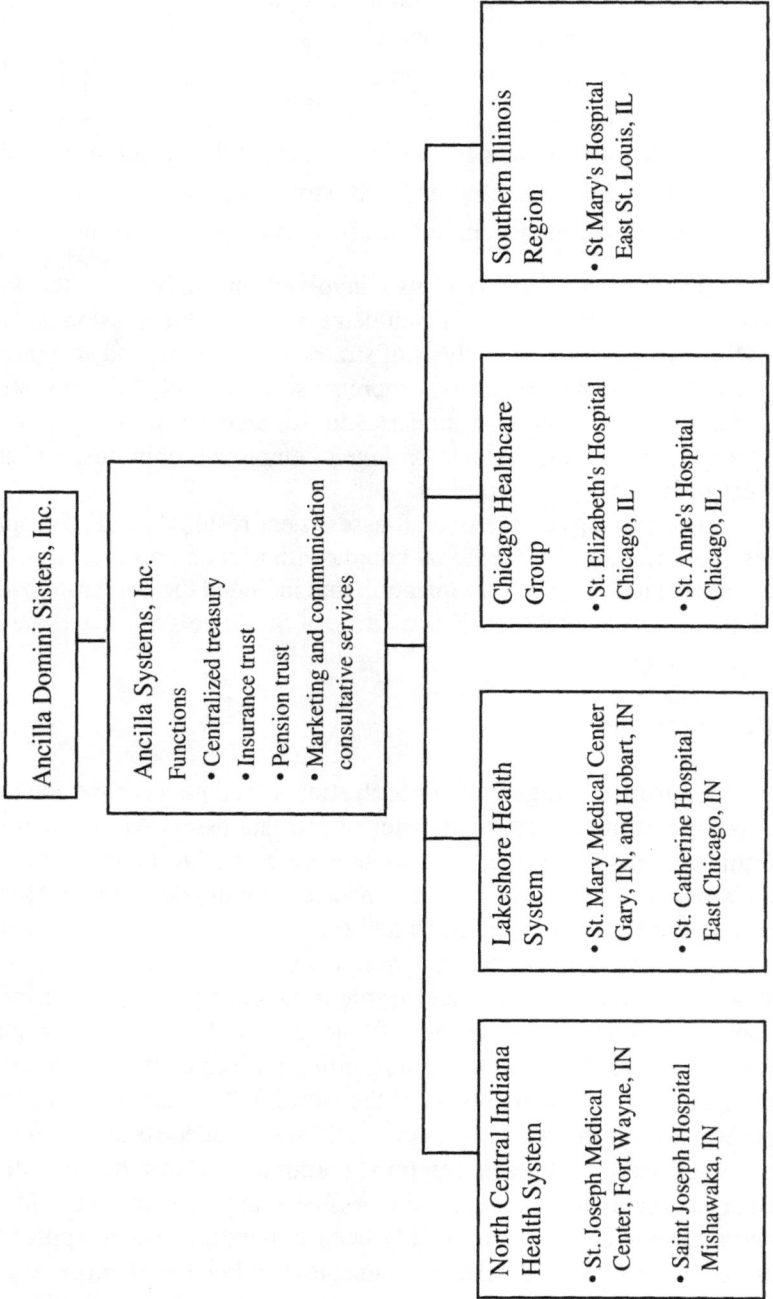

system levels and enable affiliates to more promptly respond to market needs.

Finally, and extremely critical to the success of the restructuring plan, was the implementation of management contracts. As a result of the assessment to determine the roots of the existing problems within the system, it became clear that progress toward operational and financial improvements would not be forthcoming unless governance and management roles and responsibilities were more clearly defined at the system and regional levels. More importantly, management needed to have clear authority to implement systemwide programs and objectives.

Each affiliate entered into a two-year management contract agreement with the parent corporation that called for ASI to provide general and financial management, consulting services, and executive leadership. The contract included the authority to reduce or consolidate staff, realign products and services, negotiate contracts, fix rates and extend credit, and guarantee or transfer funds to other system affiliates within previously established guidelines. The CEO of each new region was made a vice president of ASI. Under this new structure, ASI appoints the regional CEOs in consultation with the regional boards. Each CEO is part of the executive management team of ASI and participates in the development of all strategic directives and significant operational issues for the system (see Figure 3.1).

Downsizing and Closure

The downsizing of the system occurred simultaneously with the restructuring to eliminate financial risks. Initial steps in the downsizing included the divesting of St. Anne's West and the closure of St. Anne's Hospital in Chicago. The decision to divest St. Anne's West, a separate 50-bed facility in a near northwest suburb of Chicago, had been made in 1986 but had not been carried out.

At the time of the closure announcement in late August 1988, St. Anne's Hospital was losing about $1 million per month, resulting in excessive operating losses for the system. A significant portion of that loss was due to nonpayment and underpayment from Medicare and Medicaid reimbursements. While the closure decision was extremely painful to the system, the sponsor, and the community, it was critical to the process of saving the remaining institutions within the system.

The system had acquired St. Anne's West in 1981 in an effort to capture a portion of the migration of patients from St. Anne's inner-city community and in the hopes that the projected favorable payer mix would help support its inner-city sister hospital. That goal was never realized. Instead, St. Anne's West severely drained St. Anne's of its limited financial reserves. Ancilla's new leadership acted immediately to follow through on the decision to divest the facility and stop the financial drain to the system. The delay in divestiture resulted in diminishing the value of the asset, making the sale in 1987 difficult. As a result, the full value of the property was not realized.

Other Risks Eliminated

Another important step taken at this point to help eliminate risk to the system's financial viability was to convert the existing Series-C bonds for the Indiana Obligated Group (which included the five Indiana affiliates and ASI) from a variable interest rate to a fixed interest rate. That action brought the series into consistency with other existing ASI bond issues, removing the risk of both accelerated debt payment and increased debt service cost. Considerable external assistance in the areas of legal and investment banking expertise was recruited to ensure the speedy and efficient conversion. This enabled the system to take advantage of the available favorable fixed interest rates.

While these actions took place, other refinements and restructuring had been set into motion to reinforce various parts of the system. Strategies were implemented to strengthen market share at all the affiliates; following state approval, St. Anne's successful 30-bed psychiatric unit was moved to St. Elizabeth's, thereby strengthening St. Elizabeth's market share; and the system was further downsized to bring costs into line with the competition. Management was beginning to see that while the changes were difficult, they had resulted in positive strides. It was becoming apparent that a new, integrated system was emerging.

Management Refinements and Their Effects

The strategic approach and approved directives guided the reshaping of the corporate structures into four manageable entities. It also set into motion ASI's internal management restructuring. The financial, computer, operations, communications, human resources, planning, and most other corporate and affiliate departments have been examined and refined in a concentrated effort to improve the system's financial condition and achieve operational goals. New leadership at the system and regional levels is being put into place to carry out the new strategies that were established for the system in 1988. These are the achievement of financial viability; the delivery of quality service; responsiveness to regional market needs; a dedication to intense government liaison and advocacy on the local, state, and federal levels; and partnerships with other health care providers, including physician groups.

To understand Ancilla's turnaround, one must look at each of these strategies individually, understand why each was important, and view the progress made in each area.

Financial viability. This first strategy was and is crucial to both the rest of the strategies and to the system's survival. Lack of financial viability brought about the realization that complete overhaul was needed. Ancilla's new leadership had to immediately attack its financial problems on all fronts. Leadership's commitment to collect its accounts receivable, establish an aggressive monitoring system to meet daily and weekly systemwide targets, revamp its entire financial reporting system, improve cash management, and reduce administrative costs has brought substantial return to the organization in remarkable time.

Improvement in the system's cash management includes the system's restructuring of its pension plan, which had been unnecessarily overfunded. The restructuring realized an increase in net income to the system of over $20 million in 1988 with an additional $2 million anticipated in 1989. Termination of the old plan allowed the system to recoup excess funds from better-than-expected investment performance and conservative actuarial assumptions. The funds realized have been allocated to the affiliated hospitals for much needed capital reserves and have been used to pay off portions of the restructured Chicago affiliates' debt. The new plan has lowered system costs, and employees now share in investment performance. Retirement benefits are projected to be equal to or greater than under the old plan.

All business and liability insurance vehicles were restructured as well. This action has reduced the hospitals' contributions to the insurance trust, improving their cash flow. Rigorous risk management programs are being put into place.

Cash management improvements for the system also included gains from an improved investment portfolio, which the corporate restructuring has allowed to be maintained on a systemwide basis. This approach takes advantage of the total resources of the affiliates to provide funds for systemwide growth. It further eliminates unnecessary and redundant services while reducing costs. Since the inception of this approach, the annual investment yield of the cash management program has substantially exceeded that of standard Wall Street indicators.

Similarly, benefits have been realized from the creation of a centralized collection facility (CCF), established as a specific function of the corporation to perform centralized collection services for the hospitals. Accounts not collected within a certain number of days are turned over to CCF. Since the facility's inception in 1988, net revenue days for accounts receivable have dropped from a systemwide average of 94 days to 80.1 days. More than $10 million in actual cash was collected through CCF in its first year of operation.

Under the new financial strategy, the corporation also made a significant commitment to the internal audit function, expanding its capability and adding staff in 1988 to achieve corporate commitments. This resulted in more frequent and in-depth reviews of internal controls at all levels, as well as greater compliance with corporate and affiliate policies. The internal audit department also reviews all third-party reimbursement processes to ensure that cost reports are accurate, contractual receipts and allowances are properly stated, and cost reimbursement is maximized. The restructuring of this department and process reduced external audit costs by $100,000 for fiscal years 1987 and 1988.

Efforts have also been undertaken to achieve streamlined and consistent accounting and financial reporting through the establishment of more uniform key indicators for the system's reporting processes. These efforts include intense internal training and the recruitment of qualified personnel to fill key positions at the corporate and affiliate levels. The effort to improve both procedures and product costing within the hospitals and budget accountability is an example of enhancements in this area. A quarterly process has been established requiring regional management to explain variances from regional and hospital budgets to both regional boards and corporate management.

In addition, an ambitious new management information system (MIS) strategy has been implemented. The new system replaced an out-of-date and costly centralized mainframe system with three regional data centers and is now supported by more efficient IBM AS/400 minicomputers. The new MIS plan emphasizes more sophisticated and more easily maintained technology. The system supports all payroll functions, as well as patient accounting, admitting, medical records, general ledger, accounts payable, and materials management. Three regional data centers are located within the Lakeshore Health System, the North Central Indiana

Region, and the Chicago area for the Illinois facilities. The corporation maintains a data center to provide a central data base for consolidation reporting and financial monitoring. The conversion reduced staffing and operational expenses by approximately $1 million in the first year. An additional $1 million is expected to be realized during the second year of operation.

Delivery of quality service. The system's commitment to the maintenance of high quality care and efficient service required the implementation of strong internal controls and a greater effort from staff than had existed. Through the comprehensive systemwide survey project discussed above, a baseline of information has been established, feedback has been summarized, and changes and improvements are being incorporated to enhance management goals and improve quality assurance programs and offerings.

Ancilla's risk management, utilization review, and medical staff review programs have all been redesigned to provide check points and opportunities geared toward programs such as educating physicians on the necessity to reduce lengths of stay and creating improvements in resource conservation to guarantee that the system does not lose Medicare funds.

Regional market responsiveness. The structuring of each region within the system into centralized regional management teams has facilitated effective management and allowed for optimal coordination of service delivery while relating to area market responsiveness. Such responsiveness is critical to the success of the turnaround to date and continues to be important to the achievement of future goals.

Each region has developed specific programs in response to health care needs and unfilled market niches within each community. For example, programs such as older adult services and enhanced home health access have been established where none existed. The recognition and expansion of the role of the physician as partner has been incorporated into the strategy; penetration into secondary markets to offset population declines has been established as a goal and results are being realized; renovation plans, conversions to private patient rooms, and other capital improvements have been implemented, where appropriate, to maintain market viability. Partnerships with other health care providers within the regions have been sought. These examples point to but a few of the numerous regional marketing strategies that have been implemented as vital parts of the system's overall restructuring.

Government liaison and external advocacy. The system mounted an aggressive government liaison program to develop and influence legislation to change reimbursement for the support of its hospitals, which provide a disproportionate share of indigent care. This strategy recognizes that hospitals like Ancilla's are in partnership with the government and must do all within their power to change government reimbursements. As the system prepares for its third legislative year, Ancilla can point to several successes in drawing legislative and public attention to the plight of inner-city hospitals. ASI has acted as a catalyst, an educator, a grass roots advocate, and a communicator, with the various state and local hospital associations and on its own. ASI's goal has been to convey the message that the needs of the medically indigent are everyone's responsibility.

Ancilla has allocated substantial resources, both time and money, to this project and has used the services of nationally recognized advocate experts. Through Ancilla s efforts and assistance a bill was passed in Illinois that brings an additional $60 million to disproportionate-share hospitals statewide, $2 million of which will benefit ASI's two Illinois facilities. In Indiana, Ancilla's efforts helped bring about a disproportionate share adjustment; improve the state's Medicaid coverage to women and children; establish a major statewide Healthcare Study Commission to take a detailed look at the state's varied health care approaches and policies; and obtain legislatively mandated prompt payment of Medicaid claims by the state.

In another area of advocacy, Ancilla used every media opportunity surrounding the tragic closing of St. Anne's Hospital to maximize public attention to the severity of this national crisis. In staging its closure announcement, ASI included a press conference and invitation to area legislators, Catholic leaders, and other health association officials to participate in the event. The resulting coverage included every major national network news station and area affiliate. An estimated 36 million viewers had access to the story of the closing of St. Anne's. In addition, over 130 newspapers and news journals in 32 states, including all major dailies, covered this important story. As a follow-up, two major networks did in-depth feature stories on the national tragedy of hospital closings using St. Anne's as the vehicle to demonstrate the issue. In every case the story of government underfunding and the plight of our nation's poor and underserved were dramatized.

Collaboration and partnerships. In addition to the programs already cited, Ancilla has entered into joint ventures and partnerships consistent with the system's mission to fully round out the restructuring and guarantee adherence to its strategies. Throughout the system, the role of physicians is being recognized and expanded to further include these important members of the hospital family within the sphere of responsibility and authority. In Ft. Wayne, St. Joseph's has collaborated with one of the two other area major health care providers to better serve the community and eliminate the duplication of laboratory and clinical services. In the Southern Illinois Region, ASI's St. Mary's Hospital of East St. Louis is currently serving as the catalyst for a coalition of social and health care services in an attempt to create a new model for the delivery of services. It is hoped that the myriad of health care and social problems in this dramatically disadvantaged area can be addressed in partnership with the State of Illinois, the city of East St. Louis, community leaders in St. Clair County, area academic institutions, other health care providers, and human services agencies.

In Chicago, discussions are ongoing with potential partners in St. Elizabeth's Hospital's service delivery area to achieve a balance of services in what is commonly perceived as an overbedded area. Alignments with other health care providers could ultimately include a sharing of some responsibilities and authority within the St. Elizabeth's service area.

In the area served by what was the St. Anne's market, Ancilla Systems has continued its presence through physician services still operating in its professional office building and has maintained an ongoing dialogue with community groups in seeking a clinic approach to the delivery of other health care and social services for the area. The system has continued to provide the forum for exploring a series of alternative health care delivery systems to fill voids and has been instrumental in garnering the attention of community-based foundations to assist in its efforts to secure funds for the exploration of such delivery systems.

Other Key Factors

Restructuring the system to make it more responsive was essential to both the turnaround process and its implementation. Simultaneous and speedy movement in all areas was critical if the system was to get past the many and varied crises on all fronts. Outside expertise was used extensively to implement the plans for restructuring each specific area. Highly experienced consultants in such areas as finance, banking, information systems, pension conversion, information systems, cost accounting, strategic planning, human resources, advocacy, quality assurance, and risk management were brought in to augment in-house skills. This expertise enhanced major financial strengthening steps such as the establishment of CCF, the MIS conversion, and the pension plan conversion to be initiated and carried out almost simultaneously.

The Remaining Challenges

The partnership between internal staff and consultants has brought the system to where it has now redefined and reconfigured itself and its institutions into becoming more streamlined, more high tech, and more operationally efficient. As indicated earlier, all these steps combined stopped the bleeding and pumped new life into the patient. The current challenge facing leadership is one of continued refinement to ensure viability for the future.

Across the system, the strategic planning process is in high gear. The process is being approached and managed in unison toward the goal of creating an integrated medical and delivery system with emphasis on nonacute care in several regions. At this stage, markets are being examined more closely than during the initial assessment overview. This phase of examination is geared toward creating better market shares within ASI's communities of operation, defining natural markets, and seeking partnerships within each region—with physicians, other providers, and other entities. Regional planners, operating at the affiliate level and coordinated at the corporate level, are assessing population patterns and decisions are being made that consider an area's aging patterns, lifestyles, and other demographic factors. The physician has become a more integral player in the determination of programs and utilization policies, a key factor to the regional strategies developed for Ancilla Systems in the 1990s.

Other regional strategies center around a number of key thrusts, including the system's redefined identity and values; a regional component of the system's advocacy strategy to build bridges within ASI's communities to raise funds and support; stewardship patterned to develop more effective utilization of system resources and the synergies of systemness; increased emphasis on quality; and the exploration of the delivery of services outside the hospital setting.

Foundation development at each affiliate is in progress to organize programs of planned giving as well as to seek philanthropic foundation and government monies to fund unique programs in support of ASI's mission.

Regional leadership is being closely examined to ensure that the right expertise exists to reinforce the system's long-term goals and changes.

Critical to the success of the system's new design is the determination of who will direct it, both from a management and governance perspective. Flexibility is also key to the development of strategies at this stage. Whatever shape evolves for the system, it must have the flexibility to adjust itself to unpredictable challenges.

Not the least among the regional strategies being discussed is the delivery of the highest achievable standard of care, delivered in the most cost-efficient manner. To that end, extensive quality measurements will be further incorporated. Emphasis is on the best and most productive work by all individuals.

These parts of the regional emphasis all represent the remaining challenges of Ancilla's mission as its prepares itself for the future.

A Retrospective: What Worked Best and What Could Have Been Done Differently

In retrospect, one of the best actions taken in the turnaround process was the rapid decision by new leadership to immediately restructure before attempting to implement further change. Without streamlining the management and governance accountability process, subsequent successes would have been difficult if not impossible.

It can also be said that the best decisions were the most difficult. Had those decisions—like the divestiture of noncontributing assets, closing St. Anne's Hospital, and making major personnel changes—been easier to make, they might have been made earlier, and the crisis might not have reached a level that demanded immediate and sweeping action.

The success of the implementation of so many changes so rapidly and simultaneously hinged significantly on communication. That communication included dialogue with governance boards, staff, and, where necessary, external audiences.

Clearly, any large undertaking has elements that could have been improved on, and Ancilla System's turnaround is no exception. One such element that could have effected a smoother transition would have been to bring in the new management team immediately under the CEO sooner. Earlier successes on the regional level might also have been realized had the strategy to bring physicians into the process been emphasized earlier.

Finally, in hindsight, the system probably began some collaborative partnership discussions too prematurely, before Ancilla was financially viable enough to present itself as valued partner.

Leadership's Vision of the Future

Ancilla has a vision of becoming a leader in the development of regional delivery of care, having its name be synonymous with excellence, and being recognized within the industry for its managerial skills. That vision includes being perceived as an advocate in health care for the poor and disadvantaged.

Those who direct ASI today are profoundly aware of the heritage of its sponsoring congregation, the Poor Handmaids of Jesus Christ. The mission today is one of perpetuating the system's values and commitments to the compassionate care, community, quality, and stewardship that Katherine Kasper, the sponsor's foundress, began and that the system strives to achieve. This has always been the mission of the system in whatever form it has functioned. Today, this traditional commitment must be carried out in modern terms within a high-tech industry, in partnership with a laity pledged to the values of the Catholic church. That is the only way to preserve Katherine Kasper's vision. The current restructuring has prepared ASI to survive into the next century, achieve its vision of leadership, and perpetuate its values.

4

A FINANCIAL TURNAROUND

Thomas H. Rockers

Editors' Note: This turnaround necessitated the reduction of more employees than any other single turnaround described in the book. It also describes the turnaround process from a system perspective. Special attention is given to the diagnostic process an executive new to the community uses. The role of most major publics in the turnaround process is reviewed. The development of strategic plans and the importance of the strategic reallocation of resources to meet the needs of a community, not to simply contribute to the financial turnaround of an organization, is also described.

Success is never final. Failure is never fata l. It is courage that counts.

—Sir Winston Churchill

The Situation

Santa Rosa Health Care Corporation is a regional multihospital system owned and operated by the Incarnate Word Health Services, which is the parent. In early 1987, with the retirement of the chief executive officer, the board of directors of Santa Rosa Health Care Corporation believed it was necessary to bring on a CEO with the skills necessary to reposition the organization and change the corporate structure into a true regional multihospital system so as to ensure that each hospital would be responsive to its respective market. To that end, they recruited a new CEO, Thomas H. Rockers, in June 1987.

On the CEO's arrival, the situation at Santa Rosa Health Care Corporation could best be described as a great deal of commitment by a large number of good people on a course of financial disaster, if not ruin, unless strong corrective action was taken. The corporation at that time comprised four hospitals with a total of 1,118 licensed beds, a nonprofit PPO, a for-profit parent company that held two for-profit partnerships, a for-profit medical facilities corporation, and a for-profit durable medical company. The gross revenue of Santa Rosa Health Care Corporation for 1987 was about $150 million, and free care provided to the community was about $11 million.

In 1986, the corporation lost $772,000. The admissions for the corporation steadily declined from 29,000 in 1985 to a projected 17,000 in 1987. In September of 1986, the new St. Rose Hospital was opened and became operational. The length of stay for the corporation hospitals was considerably above the national norm. Market share decreased from 16 percent in 1983 to 13 percent by 1986. From 1982 to 1987, the total discharges for the corporation decreased 19.7 percent, the total number of patient days for the corporation decreased 26.3 percent, and the average daily census within the hospitals decreased 25 percent. In June 1987, financial figures showed a loss of about $1 million a month. After the final audit was completed for 1987, the total loss for the corporation was $16,102,000. Overall decrease in cash for year-end 1987 was approximately $13 million, which left a cash reserve of approximately $8 million at the start of 1988.

The four hospitals that made up Santa Rosa Health Care Corporation were all distinctly different and had a similar pattern of erosion in the marketplace, but for different reasons. Santa Rosa Hospital, the oldest of the four institutions, was originally established in 1869 and emerged as the largest Catholic hospital on one site in the United States, with approximately 1,000 licensed beds under one roof. Santa Rosa has a downtown location in a city in which one out of five families' incomes is within the federal poverty guidelines. It was perceived as seeing a higher proportion of Medicaid patients than its competing hospitals within the city. The strong, rich heritage of the Santa Rosa Hospital, one time the premier hospital in the city, had gradually eroded with a population shift to the suburbs and the creation of a medical center approximately 20 miles from the downtown location. The relocation of the county hospital from downtown to the suburbs left the downtown Santa Rosa with the perception that it was the hospital for the economically disadvantaged patient. The medical staff at Santa Rosa Hospital gradually lost support of new specialists in the community and thus lost a great deal of market share in the managed care population. The institution was a solid institution made up of good people who did not feel good about themselves and wanted desperately to recapture the quality image yet take care of the economically disadvantaged and be financially successful.

Santa Rosa Hospital was the economic driver for the corporation for a long period of time, and that continued in 1987. It had the highest volume of patients for the system and also the highest revenue and costs. It tried to be all things to all people. It had all services and tried to provide the total range of health care one would expect in a major downtown 500-bed institution; however, the average daily census was dropping rapidly from 461 per day in 1984 to no more than 300 patients at any time in 1987. The competition for the Santa Rosa downtown hospital consisted of four other downtown hospitals that were all adult institutions ranging in size from 416 occupied beds to 82 beds. The total average daily census of the five adult downtown hospitals decreased 33.7 percent from 1980 to 1986.

Santa Rosa Children's Hospital is a downtown facility with 150 licensed beds colocated with the Santa Rosa adult hospital. Children's Hospital was created in 1959. At that time, it was the only Children's Hospital in San Antonio, but over the years, as a result of the management and physician structure, Children's Hospital started to lose its own identity. It became branded as Santa Rosa as opposed to the Children's Hospital. The number of discharges steadily decreased at Children's Hospital from 7,674 in 1982 to 4,384 in 1987, a decrease of 42.9 percent. Patient days had a similar sharp decline of 29.7 percent from 1982 to 1987. The average daily census went from 134 patients in 1982 to 89 patients in 1987, a decrease of 33.6 percent. At the same time, the average length of stay for the Children's Hospital increased from 6.0 days to 7.4 days, an increase of 23.3 percent. Because of the Children's Hospital location downtown, it too began to be branded as a Medicaid children's hospital. Children's Hospital's physical plant was showing a great deal of wear and tear as well. Financial loss was constant because the Medicaid reimbursement in Texas was insufficient. The percent of Medicaid at Children's was not dissimilar to other parts of the country—about 40 percent; however, the reimbursement in Texas was bad. The majority of the free care for the Santa Rosa Health Care Corporation came through Children's patients. In 1987, that amount of free care was estimated to be approximately $9 million.

Children's Hospital's main competitor was a pediatric ward of a 20-year-old general medical-surgical hospital in the suburbs. Because of its location, the pediatric patients at that hospital were all insured; therefore, private physicians in the community were gradually being driven toward supporting that competing institution.

When Rockers came on board in 1987, one of the major issues facing Santa Rosa Health Care Corporation was a consultant's report stating the Children's Hospital should move from its downtown location out to the suburban Medical Center. That would leave only a small number of pediatric beds downtown colocated with Santa Rosa for meeting the indigent needs of the population that lived close to the Children's Hospital. Children's was really fighting for its own identity. It had no management staff of its own; it had no medical staff of its own. All concerned had a great deal of doubt about its financial viability. It had a major teaching affiliation with the University of Texas Health Science Center at San Antonio and can best be described as having no solid direction except for trying to give quality care to the patients who gravitated to its doors.

Villa Rosa Hospital is a 254-licensed-bed psychiatric facility about 15 miles from the downtown hospitals, in the Medical Center. It too had a pattern of decreased discharges from 3,061 in 1982 to 2,670 in 1987, a 12.8 percent decrease. Patient days decreased 36.7 percent over the same period, and the average daily census went from 186 in 1982 to 118 in 1987, a 36.6 percent decrease. In 1977 Villa Rosa Hospital was the only psychiatric facility in San Antonio; however, by 1987 five other for-profit psychiatric hospitals were up and operating. At one time Villa Rosa was the major source of revenue for the Santa Rosa Health Care Corporation; but by year-end 1987 its programs had deteriorated, market share was totally split with the other new entrants into the marketplace, and Villa Rosa was struggling as a psychiatric provider.

In August 1986, St. Rose Hospital and Rehabilitation Center was opened as a new 200-bed medical-surgical and rehabilitation hospital colocated with Villa Rosa in the Medical Center complex of San Antonio, Texas. St. Rose Hospital had been planned and built under the precept of cost reimbursement before diagnosis-related groups (DRGs). In 1987 total occupancy of licensed beds within the San Antonio area was 60 percent and going down. Along with the opening of the new St. Rose Hospital, Santa Rosa Health Care Corporation also built, owned, and operated a seven-story medical office building next to St. Rose Hospital. The opening of St. Rose Hospital did not provide the influx of patients that was initially anticipated. In June 1987, the office building occupancy was only 20 percent. The hospital had no identity among a cluster of seven other hospitals in the same geographic area. Daily census was at about 50 to 60 patients. The hospital originally had an obstetrics service, but after three months, there were only three deliveries and it was closed. The great promise that this new hospital would provide a revenue source in a geographic area with paying patients was not coming to fruition for the corporation. It had no medical niche and its survivability was questionable.

On arriving, the first questions the new CEO asked of the then present management team left little doubt that there was limited reliable financial information. Missing were up-to-date computerized systems of information flow. In its place was a highly centralized bureaucratic management structure that did not allow for the hospitals' separate identities or the identification of institutional markets. The board of directors was not as informed as they should have been. The mission was strong; the tradition was strong. The management structure was defective and highly bureaucratic. Confidence was totally lacking.

Since the Santa Rosa Health Care Corporation was part of a bond indenture with the Incarnate Word Health Services, the parent corporate office was very concerned about financially turning Santa Rosa around. The entire system was financially jeopardized by carrying the $50 million debt the Santa Rosa Health Care Corporation held.

Review of the Situation After 18 Months

The first 18 months were marked by total corporate reorganization into a multidivisional hospital organization with the creation of three hospital governing boards for the different markets to be served. Massive change at the senior management level and the creation of a new management structure allowed for decentralized line authority and management at the individual hospital level with a CEO at the St. Rose and Villa Rosa Hospitals, a CEO at Santa Rosa Hospital, and a CEO at the Children's Hospital. Central corporate staff support in finance, strategic resources and planning, and institutional advancement was created.

Five strategic plans were developed: one for the whole Santa Rosa Health Care Corporation, one for Villa Rosa Hospital, one for St. Rose Hospital and Rehabilitation Center, one for Santa Rosa Hospital, and one for Children's Hospital. This process involved over 200 physicians, board members, and staff. The information system of the organization had a new direction and focus. The number of employees in the overall corporation was decreased by about 35 management positions and 300 full-time equivalents (FTEs). Children's Hospital was relicensed as a free-standing hospital for reimbursement purposes, and Villa Rosa Hospital was relicensed as a free-standing psychiatric institution to compete with the other free-standing licensed psychiatric hospitals. A total management training program was developed to ensure that all new managers practice the same management philosophy. New contracts were negotiated with all managed care providers within the City of San Antonio. The occupancy of the medical office building colocated with St. Rose went from 20 percent to 98 percent. Psychiatric programs at Villa Rosa Hospital changed from a medical model to a program model.

Three individual medical staffs were created: one for the Santa Rosa Hospital, one for Children's Hospital, and one for St. Rose and Villa Rosa Hospitals. The total number of admissions for the corporation increased for the first time in five years. Admissions in 1988 increased by 82, while the total marketplace continued to decrease. Market share therefore increased as well for the first time in seven years. A renewed spirit of success and fulfillment permeated all levels. The medical staffs took ownership of the situation and implemented quality assurance mechanisms that decreased the length of stay significantly and altered the patterns of practice of a large number of physicians, forcing some physicians to leave the facility. Children's hospital board, medical staff, and management committed to remaining downtown.

Most importantly in 1988, the corporation's hospital operations showed a profit of $184,000. For the overall corporation, the loss was reduced from $16 million in 1987 to $1.3 million.

Process Used to Understand Organizational Issues

The CEO of Santa Rosa Health Care Corporation, coming into a new situation and not knowing the exact magnitude of all problems, took the approach of first and foremost listening hard to as many people as possible with the intent of understanding the marketplace reality of the San Antonio area. The CEO decided do an extensive marketing analysis by personal interview to discern how physicians, both those utilizing the facilities and those who did not, as well as the board members viewed the situation. That process took approximately six months. Every day, contact was made with at least four physicians or business people within the community, asking the same questions: Tell me how you think Santa Rosa Health Care Corporation can better serve the community? What did we do wrong? What did we do right? How can we improve? Will you help me? After one month of this type of interviewing and also asking questions internally for data and personal opinion, the CEO knew that the major issue, financial viability, could not wait.

Audits from previous years and financials available initially indicated that there was enough capital to allow the CEO time to understand and set direction for this system. By the end of the second month on the job, it became clear that without swift action by the end of 1987 the corporation would be financially insolvent as early as mid-1988. Thus, the immediate situation had to be diagnosed.

To fix the short-term problems, the new CEO decided on an organizational form and management structure for the multihospital corporation that would not only meet short-term needs but also be compatible with long-term strategy. Recruitment to fill the vacant management positions began as fast as possible, first recruiting a CEO for the new St. Rose Hospital while simultaneously recruiting a senior vice-president for Finance, and other key senior management and CEO. It was imperative to have the right people on board before major cost cutting or layoffs could take place. Strategic decisions were made first; detailed decisions followed.

The analytical process undertaken was from a system approach and not an individual institution approach. The first requirement was to find out as much as possible about the marketplace and the economics of the San Antonio area. What were the major drivers? What was the history? What was the future? What were the demographics? Where was the growth pattern? What were the capabilities of all the competing institutions? Was there a systemized approach to health care within the San Antonio area? What was the position of managed care in the San Antonio marketplace? Most importantly, what was the best way to stop the hemorrhaging of cash, get costs down, and at the same time get the organization on the road to acquiring new patient business and take this business away from other institutions? After two months there was no more time for diagnosis. Swift corrective action began.

To make sure that all decisions made from a strategic standpoint were done with the most knowledge possible of the marketplace and individual hospital needs and capabilities, Santa Rosa Health Care Corporation embarked on a major strategic planning process with an outside consulting firm, Cambridge Research Institute. This firm was selected because of their capability of involving and committing people quickly. The corporation had to set its strategic plans as quickly as possible to make sure the long-term viability of the corporation was solid while at the same time taking corrective actions to solve short-term financial problems.

The strategic planning process had major issues to address and directions to set. The process had to answer the question of the proper size and location of all of the hospital facilities of the Santa Rosa Health Care Corporation. Were they optimally located? Were additional units needed?

What was the size of the regional market? Were the institutions in the correct regional market niches? What was the best approach for this system in San Antonio? Should all hospitals be full service medical-surgical hospitals? Was the corporation coordinating as much involvement of the physicians as possible?

The strategic planning process became operational in December 1987 with a completion deadline of May 1988. The strategic planning process was separated into distinct phases or components to carefully analyze every part of the system's business. The first component required the corporation itself to examine how it should be organized. What was the major business of the corporation going to be? Should it continue diversification efforts? What was the role of the corporation? What was the role of its subsidiaries?

In total, five strategic plans were established. One was developed for the corporation, and the second strategic plan focused on Santa Rosa Hospital as a distinct unit. The Children's Hospital was also outlined as a strategic element with planning targeting the medical staff. Although St. Rose and Villa Rosa Hospitals were organized administratively as one unit, two strategic plans were developed. Determining marketplace realities for medical-surgical services and rehabilitation in the market where St. Rose was located required a separate plan. The psychiatric hospital, Villa Rosa, had a separate plan to diagnose the situation within the regional psychiatric marketplace. Other general strategic needs identified were the capability of capital generation and the general needs for capital long-term, as well as possible improvement in corporate profitability in the marketplace. The relationships among the University of Texas Health Science Center at San Antonio, Santa Rosa Health Care Corporation, and the hospital divisions also needed to be addressed.

Most important, however, a strategy needed to be developed to rebuild market share and create a take-away strategy for the San Antonio marketplace. Finally, the long-term position of the Santa Rosa Health Care Corporation with relationship to managed health care in the San Antonio area needed to be determined. These then became the long-range strategic questions to be answered in the process that followed so that the long-term decisions made over five years could include as much input and direction as possible.

These two approaches then became the process for understanding the organizational problems. The first was short-term. The right people needed to be in the right management positions as quickly as possible to assist in that process. The second phase was the long-term process of understanding the marketplace and the evolving of a comprehensive strategic plan involving over 200 people, most of whom were valued customers or physicians.

Approach and Implementation of the Various Components of the Santa Rosa Health Care Corporation

Role of the Board

The board of directors of the Santa Rosa Health Care Corporation played a vital role in the financial turnaround. First and foremost, the directors gave their full support to the new CEO and his efforts to develop plans for success and gave him the latitude to take any action necessary to change management personnel to accomplish the overall goals of the corporation. They also supported the governance restructuring that created three new hospital division boards, including decreasing the board size from 17 down to 10.

Role of Top Management

In this financial turnaround the role of top management was twofold: (1) The right top management had to be in place to help make decisions on cost reduction with the proper management being held accountable for making the decisions on FTE reductions as well as other costs. (2) Senior management had to be in place for the strategic plans to be developed and then implemented. Once these two functions were accomplished by top management, there was total commitment to both cost reduction and the implementation of the strategic plans. The role of top management continues to be to ensure that the corporation's goals and objectives permeate all divisions and that all divisions work in unison to accomplish the corporation's overall strategy.

Role of the Medical Staff and Its Leadership

The role of the medical staff in this turnaround was unique. In late 1987, there was one medical staff for all the hospitals. The medical staff leadership

1. encouraged the new CEO and his management team to decentralize as much of the decision making as possible and create three distinct medical staffs in place of one,
2. helped implement many of the cost reductions on personnel throughout the organization because they could see the inefficiencies built up over the years of bureaucracy,

3. totally supported a redirection with quality as the basis for all decision making and the process required, and

4. were totally involved in the strategic repositioning of each of the hospitals and were partners in developing the strategic plans for each institution.

Their support in the creation of the three additional hospital governing boards was crucial; the restructuring increased physician representation from two on the corporate board to a total of ten overall on the hospital and the corporate governing boards. The medical staffs became very supportive after the new CEO and management team made them part of the process and promised that they would be involved in decision making. Because of that involvement, they were highly supportive of the overall process.

Role of the Employees

The general employees were very supportive during this transition process. Although approximately 350 FTE positions were eliminated in late 1987 and early 1988, employees knew that reorganization was necessary. It was generally recognized that there were a lot of unnecessary positions. Remaining employees recognized the need to continue to work hard and become more involved in the day-to-day running of the institution for the hospitals to survive. While it is always hard to pinpoint exactly the feelings of employees during this turnaround, in Santa Rosa Health Care Corporation's case the increased involvement of employees during the process created an atmosphere of pride in being associated with a growing and vibrant organization as opposed to an organization having trouble with its direction. In 1987 and 1988, all employees received cash Christmas bonuses for their efforts. Benefit plans were improved, and salaries were raised to meet competitive standards in the community, resulting in the best year ever for recruiting nursing personnel to fill vacant positions.

Role of Key Committees

All committees were important, but most crucial in the turnaround was the President's Task Force. This group of five trustees of the Santa Rosa Health Care Corporation board met monthly with the CEO, provided a sounding board, and gave additional counsel and input to the CEO before final recommendations were made to the corporate board. This committee, which existed for about 11 months, acted until the final reorganization was approved at the corporate level, when an executive committee of the board was formed in its place.

Other key committees were those involved in the strategic planning process for the four hospitals, as well as the corporation's strategic planning committee. These committees gave a great deal of time, effort, and input developing the necessary strategy in each of the institutions, as well as guiding the overall corporation board and management in developing key strategies for the corporation.

Role of Materials Management

Materials management was identified early on as a key cost saving element. To that end, nationally known consultants analyzed the laundry system as well as the overall materials management system. The consultants' recommendations resulted in the following: (1) Overall inventories of the corporation were too high; therefore, programs began to reduce inventories throughout the corporation, resulting in a first year's savings of about $308,000 for inventory reduction and projected $300,000 in the second year. (2) A central warehousing operation was instituted, with full implementation in April 1989. All warehousing is now off-site for the four hospitals, and all purchasing is centralized throughout the corporation. The materials management function continues to be a key cost reduction program for the corporation with long-term savings exceeding $2 million after all departmental changes and modifications throughout the corporation were computed by year-end 1989.

External Factors Affecting the Turnaround

In mid-1987, the corporation's relationship with managed health care companies in the San Antonio area was hostile. By the end of 1988, after all new contracts were drawn up and new business secured, the health maintenance organization and PPO business for the corporation increased 77 percent as a result of aggressive positive efforts. The end of 1988 showed a 10 percent admission rate for all managed health care as contrasted with a mid-1987 percentage of 3 to 4 percent. This factor had the greatest financial impact on new admissions and also positioned the corporation across the city as a strong long-term player in the marketplace.

Remaining Challenges to Complete and Improve the Corporation

The remaining challenges that face Santa Rosa Health Care Corporation are predictable.

1. A constant vigilance regarding the quality of medical staff serving all the institutions. Competent, skilled physicians must be willing partners of our organization. Physicians must be empowered to make changes, and management must be committed to attentively listening and to creatively helping to solve physicians' problems.

2. A constant vigilance regarding cost. The corporation's costs have been significantly reduced; however, a great deal more can and must be done to maintain this corporation in an environment where fixed prices from both the federal government and local commercial insurers are the norm and not the exception.

3. The implementation of an computerized information network. All information should be based on cost, and volumes should be directly related to reality and not projections. This information must be swiftly turned around.

4. The biggest challenge for the corporation: securing additional capital resources (without incurring any more debt on the parent Incarnate Word Health Services bond) to recapitalization the downtown facilities. The downtown facilities need approximately $20 million worth of reinvestment into mechanical, electrical, and plumbing systems over the next five years. This refurbishing will ensure continued survival of the Children's Hospital and the down-sized adult facility. The downtown facilities as well as the Northwest facilities also need capital improvements to become more outpatient driven and additional capital for high technology specialty areas.

If these challenges are satisfactorily met, the entire corporation will be on its way to strategically redirecting each of its programs to meet the needs of the San Antonio community, into the early 1990s and through the year 2000. The important issue is not simply financial turnaround but the long-term strategic reallocation of resources to meet the needs of the San Antonio community.

Hindsight

One always wishes there was more time to communicate better with affected employees, medical staff, and the public during change, but with the heavy monthly losses being incurred, the time to communicate the necessity and reasons for change did not exist, unfortunately.

One always learns from the experience of others. What can be gleaned from these experiences is that flexibility is required to understand that the solution for each of the four institutions is different. This flexibility to modify thinking assists in relating to a psychiatric institution versus a children's hospital versus a medical-surgical hospital. This is always the challenge of a multihospital organization, but in a turnaround it becomes paramount that those differences manifest themselves so that true strategic change can be accomplished, meeting the needs of the marketplace each institution is serving.

> Nothing is constant but change! All existence is a perpetual flux of "being and becoming"!
> —Ernst Heinrich Haeckel, German biologist

5

MANAGING A TURNAROUND:
FROM CONFUSION TO CONSENSUS

Mark E. Celmer

Editors' Note: The chapter describes numerous turnaround tactics and provides guidelines for leadership and people management in a turnaround. The
use of retreats and education is thoroughly described, and the changes in
management structure necessary to effectively complete the turnaround are
also considered. The chapter presents a simple operational and business plan
for a hospital turnaround and a basic outline of critical factors in improving
the financial viability of the organization.

Background and History

From a managerial perspective, an organization needs to continually
reassess its mission and vision. The purpose of this chapter is to document
some essential steps necessary for an organization that needs a breath of
fresh air to step back and reanalyze its mission and purpose. The subtitle,
"From Confusion to Consensus," is not intended to be derogatory but is
merely an effort to highlight what can quickly happen when a health care
organization falls into a level of complacency or attempts to cling to the
past and rely too heavily on previous successes. Although this article
focuses on a quiet suburban community hospital in a northern suburb of
Buffalo, New York, I have drawn on many other career observations to
equitably distribute some of my criticisms of common managerial and CEO
pitfalls.

In my opinion, DeGraff Memorial Hospital is not unique. In many community-based private institutions, management, when faced with a drastically changing external environment, attempts to maintain the status quo and cling to past accomplishments. The net affect in our current health care environment is crippled decision making at all levels within the organization.

The primary purpose in documenting this managerial approach is to help explain the financial and organizational turnaround of a hospital that, within the past few years, has been plagued with more crises than most other hospitals will see in decades. The turnaround at DeGraff can be summarized in a quote from Niccolo Machiavelli:

> There is nothing more difficult to take in hand, more perilous to conduct, or more uncertain in its success, than to take the lead in the introduction of a new order of things.

On my return to DeGraff in 1983, I inherited a fine and generally reputable institution that, by and large, was ten years behind the times.

Preliminary Steps

The Targeted Goals

In my discussions with the executive committee regarding the opportunity to return to DeGraff as its president and CEO, the board through the members of the finance committee, had delineated a broad mandate to the previous administration to address its organizational paralysis. This was the first time in DeGraff's history that the board demonstrated a level of concern and understanding that the health care environment was indeed changing and that, organizationally, DeGraff lacked the corporate flexibility and performance measurements to respond within the marketplace. In this context, the finance committee established the following written policy statement:

> The environment—political, economic, and social—in which the health industry and DeGraff Memorial Hospital as a part of that industry function, has changed drastically in recent years. Continued rapid and structural change is to be anticipated . . . it is essential that our management approach to our new environment be defined, structured in a flexible manner, and periodically evaluated.

On the basis of the above mandate, it was clear that on my return to DeGraff, the administration had to take the lead in presenting to the board a plan of objectives, a strategic plan, a financial plan, and a method of determining performance and productivity that could be easily measured and evaluated. In essence, the board sensed that the organization had to respond quickly, but as a lay group, they did not know precisely how to finesse the organization through its fiscal and demographic changes. Once again, with all due respect to the board of directors, as a voluntary lay group, it should not be its responsibility to make these organizational and daily operational decisions. Their responsibility is to set policy, to review the overall goals and objectives of the organization, and to make that organization accountable. I view the board as a managerial resource. Its members should be in-house consultants who bring particular talents and experience to the process of setting organizational directions. They should not be mired in the day-to-day issues.

Step One: Establish Organizational Accountability

As the CEO, one must be willing to take risks and establish accountability at virtually every level of the organization. In my opinion, this starts with the board of directors. Just as the CEO's and the CFO's performance is judged in the annual audit and management letter, all levels of the organization must be objectively evaluated, including the board, medical staff, top and middle management, and staff employees.

All too often the board is not held accountable for how it sets policy and overall institutional priorities. Almost without deviation, this lack of accountability creates an imbalance between the board and the CEO. If accountability includes the board of trustees, however, conflict and problem resolution becomes a smooth and orderly process. By setting clear goals and objectives for the board and evaluating their performance regularly, the administration has good documentation of any commitments it makes.

For example, if the board mandates that the administration establish a flexible organization and commits to that operational objective in writing, it would be hard pressed to bind the CEO's hands from establishing a corporate restructuring effort that clearly addresses this mandate and ensures success. The board therefore must be willing to identify its goals and objectives for the administration, the medical staff, and the department in committing to a results-oriented process with individuals to be held accountable for the successes and failures.

Step Two: Commit

Once the board and the CEO and administration have committed to the targeted goals, the CEO must be willing to take risks and make decisions that are timely, necessary, and appropriate. I have seen many CEOs who have mastered the fine art of procrastination. Put another way, some CEOs (and boards) suffer a terminal disease for which there is no DRG: the paralysis of analysis. Many CEOs get buried in a morass of problems when they delay decision making and risk taking too long, at the expense of themselves and their organizations. The successful and seasoned leader knows almost instinctively which decisions to buy time with and which decisions must be made spontaneously. By and large, the decisions that need to be made spontaneously have a higher percentage of error. On the other hand, decisions not made often have a much higher expense associated with them. Here again, the seasoned leader can quickly identify an error, be accountable for it, and promptly correct it.

In addition, if targeted goals have been established at virtually every level of the organization and is explicitly stated that all levels of the organization will be held accountable for their areas of responsibility, the CEO has almost carte blanche with those decisions critical to survival. The message cannot be stressed more adamantly: Commit!

Step Three: Compassion

I use the term *compassion* as a play on words to bridge the gap between commitment (the need to master the art of decision making) and a true passion for your work ethics and institutional values. I have never known a CEO to get into trouble with his or her organization, be it the board, medical staff, community, or others, if he or she maintained integrity, honesty, commitment for action, and, perhaps most importantly, a passion for the organization's success. In tandem two underlying principles must motivate decision making and organizational success. First, the successful CEO must be willing to take more than his or her share of the blame and less than his or her share of the credit. And secondly, the CEO cannot have a personal goals of high visibility or self-aggrandizement.

Step Four: Political Savvy

It's extremely important for the CEO and other key members of the managerial staff to analyze their political connections and savvy every 12 to 18 months. The CEO must engage in a degree of introspection to continually analyze his or her own performance. Unfortunately, the old adage, "it's lonely at the top," takes on additional meaning when one realizes that the successful CEO (who maintains modesty and humility) is also deprived of the subtle pats on the back that are critical to sustained motivation and morale. The CEO must evaluate his or her own successes and failures and the degree to which the CEO has assisted decision making elsewhere within the organization. For example, a CEO who has won many battles yet lost too many wars must be prepared to frequently analyze his or her political savvy. If not, he or she should not be overly surprised if the board of directors facilitates an abrupt change in his or her career. Additionally, a CEO who lacks political finesse and cannot communicate to the medical staff leadership in a way that perpetuates win-win decisions will be overwhelmed by weekend golf games at the country club with attorneys, physicians, public accountants, and board members. Finally, the successful and seasoned CEO must know when to fight and when not to and how to get the political sharks to attack each other rather than himself or herself. In essence, don't bleed.

Step Five: Be Driven for Success

To conclude the background primer of how to succeed and turn confusion into consensus, in addition to having commitment and passion, the CEO must be driven for the overall success and reputation of others, never for his or her own personal gain. The rewards will come and in fact do come in financial and career opportunities when the organization as a whole has benefited from your leadership ability. Related to the need to be driven by the success of others are the many egos that the CEO must continually stroke. Board members will rally behind a CEO when they have been given credit for the overall success of the organization, and physicians will support a CEO who has made it easier for them to practice quality medicine and enhance their earnings.

In the past, the CEO was the liaison between the board and the organized medical staff. All too often the CEO was pulled in different directions by factions within the organization, embroiled in adversarial conflicts, and accused of being antiphysician. With all the marketing, strategic planning, and the other activities required of today's CEO, the successful administrator is one who converts all decisions into win-win-win decisions. In essence, the CEO must "take the lead in the introduction of a new order of things." The CEO must build an entire management team behind the organization that consists of board members, physicians, top and middle management, and employees. He or she must also make it as easy as possible for the medical staff to adapt to the external forces that are quickly changing beyond their control.

As this industry continues to change, physicians can become extremely depressed, angry, and antagonistic toward federal, state, and local government mandates. The administrator must ensure legal compliance and is thus put into an adversarial position with the medical staff clinging to the status quo. Therefore, in addition to being driven for success, the successful CEO must draw on every available resource to help physicians understand how the new systems works and how they can make the best of difficult times given the CEO's and physicians dependence on each other for survival.

Planning: The Formula

The Operational Plan

Briefly stated, operational planning is an approach or formula by which short- and long-term business strategies are identified, key components are provided with (and contribute to the development of) a road map to follow, and total accountability for performance is both established and measured.

As I mentioned above, when a new CEO takes the helm, he or she must identify from the very start the organization's needs and what the CEO must accomplish. Simultaneously, the CEO must determine and commit to an approach; get the consensus and support of the board; and then stick to it, evaluate it periodically, and adjust it only when necessary and with full disclosure. Many administrators start off with all the right intentions in setting their modus operandi but completely lose their effectiveness when they deliberately or inadvertently conceal changes in their approach. When this happens, the CEO completely loses consistency, commitment (from others), understanding (from all), and, perhaps most damaging, credibility. It bears emphasizing that I have seen many capable managers lose their momentum by forgetting to follow through or by changing their approach without letting those responsible be fully aware of the changes. When this happens, those responsible for the follow-through and action plans become confused and disoriented, and the CEO can hardly hold them accountable for compliance with a new set of targets and a new process when they haven't been properly nurtured.

Exhibit 5.1 presents a formula for an operational plan that can provide the entire organization with a clear and concise statement of the annual objectives of the board, administration, and medical staff, providing the cadence to which the rest of the department within the organization must take their lead. (Exhibit 5.2 is a sample operational plan based on that formula.) The operational plan therefore serves as the heart beat of operational objectives, priorities, and identified opportunities for the three key components within the organization. Once the departmental managers clearly understand what it is the administration is attempting to achieve within the operational (or business) plan, they can focus their own organizational and departmental needs around those of the top policy makers. They can then set their goals and objectives around the core position of the organization and assume responsibility and accountability for investigation, implementation, or deletion as appropriate throughout the business plan year. It is also important to set timetables for actions so that the organization has continued momentum throughout the year. More discussion follows on the importance of the business plan.

Setting Organizational Goals

The establishment of organizational goals begins with the board and is followed by the setting of administrative goals and objectives that are coterminous with those of the medical staff. These goals must permeate the rest of the organization. Of crucial importance in the establishment of organizational goals is to target completion dates and timetables for action and reporting back through the administrative channels and responsibilities. Timetables should be considered in terms of quarters or, if possible, months. Regardless of the attempt to target completion times, the entire process would fail miserably if the administration did not mandate that this entire effort be continually evaluated and that written reports of the status of the operational planning objectives be submitted through the associate hospital directors or vice presidents. Keep in mind that the crucial element in turning an organization around is accountability. To reiterate the point

Exhibit 5.1   Formula for an Operational or Business Plan

Step 1:   State the goal or target.

Step 2:   Identify all the critical success factors for each goal projected.

Step 3:   List the action steps required to implement the program contemplated, and identify the appropriate individuals to take on the component responsibility.

Step 4:   Predetermine the methodology for evaluating and measuring the efforts and outcomes of the program.

Exhibit 5.2 Sample Operational Plan

Goal

A plan for the financial solvency of the DeGraff Memorial Hospital

Critical Success Factors

1. Increase in patient and outpatient volume; decrease costs and expenses.
2. Improve cash flow.
3. Ally or consolidate services.
4. Generate revenue.
5. Recruit primary and subspecialty physicians.

Action Steps

1. Carefully monitor physician utilization patterns throughout the hospital.
2. Monitor departmental productivity.
3. Address financial systems (e.g., billing, collection, data processing procedures).
4. Initiate joint planning efforts with Niagara Falls Memorial Medical Center.
5. Identify new services to improve gross and net revenues and improve institutionwide marketing efforts.
6. Successfully recruit primary care and subspecialty practitioners.

Evaluation and Measurement

Monthly operational reports to the board of directors (i.e., financial, administrative and clinical)

---

made above, it would be a terrible mistake to change the rules without communicating the change to the people involved. The responsibility for reporting completion, status, or changes to prescribed timetables is crucial to the overall effort to hold individuals fully accountable.

Setting the Long-Range Plan

Unfortunately, all too often long-range plans are nothing more than thick reports that identify new opportunities and that, once completed, get put on a shelf and forgotten. There are other reasons why long-range plans fail to become dynamic and fluid working documents to guide the establishment of the business plan and future organizational opportunities. These reasons include the fact that many are projected too far into the future, well beyond any individual or group's ability to forecast. Another common reason is that the long-range plan becomes too focused on one major project, be it the establishment of a medical office building or adding inpatient beds. Yet another failure relates to the fact that research has not been done well enough in advance nor comprehensively enough to support misguided goals. Lastly and perhaps most important, long-range planning efforts fail because the goals and targets are assumed to be panacea for ensuring the organization's future and because consultants and long-range planning committees conceive of the conclusions before the real managerial work has been done.

There is a straightforward way to avoid these common pitfalls. Organizations should set realistic goals for a maximum of three years. The advantage of this limit is that it allows the organization to change. Each year, while the organization is working to fulfill a given set of long-range goals, the administration is making projections for a new third year. One is always both working on the current year's planning objectives and monitoring compliance with those implemented in previous years. Again, the feedback loop in ongoing monitoring and accountability become critical. This effort enlarges as the organization diversifies and has a broader base of business opportunities and there is more to manage. In addition, in evaluating past years' progress through a flexible and dynamic long-range planning program, one cannot assume that all of the progress and new programs will live on in perpetuity. Eventually, one must change the program again and set out to decertify or discontinue programs that either have become obsolete or are no longer cost beneficial (see below).

It is extremely important that the top management of the organization motivate the board and the long-range planning committee to have a series of new services and markets continuously under consideration and under development. Services already in existence should be closely analyzed, and markets should be reassessed to see if they should be divested by virtue of their unprofitability or the inability to be all things to all people. One should consider which might be more successful as a joint venture with another health facility. In summary, the establishment of long-range objectives requires a keen and sometimes clairvoyant management impetus to move the board along in establishing three-year targets. Never assume that the mere projection of a business opportunity must result in implementation. The analysis of the strategic plan must determine which business opportunities should be pursued and which should be deleted or at least deferred.

Strategic Plan

As stated above, long-range planning is useless if it lacks the basic underlying premise of accountability. Long-range plans fail and sit on a shelf to collect dust because the top leadership of the organization consciously or unconsciously becomes complacent with the process. In my opinion, it is a direct responsibility of the CEO to make sure that the long-range planning process is just that—a process. To carry out the targeted objectives and business opportunities identified in the long-range plan, a systematic means of investigating each of the individual components to determine their business value to the organization's overall mission is needed. That system is the strategic plan. The strategic plan must be tied to the long-range plan, and it must be a consistently applied formula to test the business opportunities outlined in the long-range plan.

For example, every member of the long-range planning committee of the board, and for that matter every board member, is aware that all new business initiatives identified each year within the long-range planning process must be analyzed according to the strategic planning outline in Exhibit 5.3. In brief, the individual objective is restated, including the definition of the objective and justification. Then a prospectus that includes an external analysis, an internal analysis, a quantitative study, implementation, and finally an evaluation (review and assessment) must be submitted to the board for their input and ultimate decision. Therefore, the strategic plan becomes the administrator's opportunity to present *go* or *no go* decisions for the board. As discussed in the section above on the long-range planning process, one cannot assume that every projected business opportunity will in fact be implemented. The strategic planning effort uncovers all the variables to determine the legitimacy of entering into a joint venture or business opportunity. Often times, the decision is to delete a business objective or defer it to another year. Remember, the three-year long-range plan presumes that the board continues to write annual operational plans and objectives using the current long-range planning year as a basis for setting objectives and the business plan for the future.

Exhibit 5.3 Strategic Planning Outline

    I.   Objective (restate in the executive summary)
        A. Definition
        B. Justification

    II.   External Analysis (provide a written justification)
        A. Environmental study
        B. Market study

    III. Internal Analysis (be certain you can control it)
        A. Service capabilities
        B. Corporate structure

    IV. Quantitative Study (be certain you can afford it)
        A. Financial objectives
        B. Financial commitment
        C. Return on investment

    V.   Implementation (be certain you can run and manage it)
        A. Process
        B. Time frame
        C. Program management

    VI. Evaluation (cover your actions): Review and assessment

---

Give Managers the Tools

Many institutions do not provide managers with the necessary tools to implement their action plans (the business or operational plan). Setting organizationwide goals is an effort in futility unless the organization has the proper budgeting and responsibility reporting in place and the leadership regularly reviews them. To hold departments or managers accountable, the CEO must first give them every opportunity to produce results. Once they understand what the objectives are and are given an opportunity to analyze their own area of expertise and set their departmental business plan, they must have every opportunity of cost accounting that the board demands of the CEO.

    One final comment on operational or business planning is that only those plans and objectives that can realistically be tied to the operational and capital budgeting process should be proposed to the board of trustees for their ultimate approval. For example, the board could give priority to monitoring the organizational effectiveness under a DRG method of reimbursement, but unless virtually every expense and revenue center within the hospital knows and understands the income and expenses under this reimbursement mandate, the administration cannot possibly hold them accountable for their departmental efficiency. The organization must provide the departmental leadership with monthly statistical information, a cost accounting system (including but not limited to income and expense statements by cost center, and productive and nonproductive hours), a staffing plan, and variance reports to allow them the opportunity to control their component of the business.

What to Do Before Accepting the Job

Throughout this entire approach, one aspect of management cannot be overemphasized: accountability. However, there is an important secret in holding virtually every level of the organization accountable. The CEO must have enough self-confidence in and commitment to his or her ability and talent. He or she must negotiate the right to set his or her own administrative goals in the employment agreement. If the CEO is at all timid or too motivated or attracted to the job offer, he or she will have an uphill climb. The CEO will end up attempting to hold the board accountable after the fact. However, if the CEO establishes clearly with the full board before accepting the job that he or she will consistently and regularly report to the full board progress, delays, successes, and failures but also that the board will be evaluated on its successes, failures, and progress, then a rewarding accountability process is established.

All too often, the ultimate evaluation of the CEO's performance is reduced to a discussion surrounding a salary adjustment that coincides with the annual performance evaluation of the organization as audited by the outside accountants. I feel strongly the board should not tie administration salaries to the outcome of the external audit. The board must commit to the same level of accountability and reporting relationship to the CEO as the CEO commits to them. This demand is not as ominous as it might sound since, in all candor, the CEO is going to be doing all the legwork for the board anyway. Yet if each committee of the board does not support the CEO, the CEO must be willing to stand up and tell the board that their lack of support or inaction on a business opportunity can stifle the future success and viability of that organization. Of course the laypeople on most hospital boards want to keep the community hospital in the forefront of health care delivery, but the hospital must function as a business, and survival is critical. If the CEO intends to stay viable as the leader of the organization, he or she must be certain to lead the board so that it is following the same process the CFO is, as outlined above.

The other essential element in the days before the arrival of the new CEO is to get the executive committee and president of the board to agree with a written and acceptable conflict of interest policy as a mandate of the board executive committee. Any CEO who accepts a position in an institution that does not have a concise board and organizational policy statement with regard to conflicts of interest is, in my opinion, committing managerial suicide. In a $10, $50, or $100 million business, the CEO and board must agree that nothing is sacred. It is perfectly acceptable for the CEO to be identified as the catalyst behind the establishment or reaffirmation of the conflict of interest statement; however, this issue is so crucial to agree on before the CEO takes the job that the chairman of the board, or at a minimum the treasurer, should be the one to report it to the full board. On the issue that nothing is sacred, that includes the banking institution with which the hospital or other organizational entities conduct business, external legal support (firm or firms), investment advisors, certified public accountants, and inside contracts such as emergency room, radiology, laboratory, and others.

The CEO should be sensitive to the fact that the board's prior decisions were probably prudent ones at the time. Part of the finesse of managing change is not to alienate board members who feel they made good decisions in the best interests of the hospital. The CEO must present to the board that all contracts and arrangements will be reviewed within a given time frame and that although decisions reached previously were right and proper at the time, different decisions might be necessary for the institution to progress. The successful CEO can finesse this arrangement in such a way to give the board and those responsible for earlier decisions pride of authorship in those decisions. Be sincere and give them all due credit, but at the same time, be certain that all decisions are carefully reviewed and changed if necessary.

Internal Management: At the Top

Medical Staff Relations

I have never known a viable institution with a reputable and competent CEO who did not earn the respect of the medical staff. The question is how difficult is it and how long it takes to earn that respect and how much blood shed is necessary for the medical staff to come around to the CEO's organizational philosophy. Most individual physicians and medical staffs who are attempting to function under our current climate of change and loss of autonomy attempt to cling to the status quo. This resistance is natural, and the CEO must be sensitive to it. The ultimate success of the CEO in earning the respect of the medical staff is a function of the CEO's ability to turn every decision into a united win-win opportunity. The organizational philosophy should perpetuate win-win-win opportunities, placing the benefits to the patient and community first, followed by the organization and physician. The interrelationship of the board, medical staff, and administration is one of pure, unadulterated politics, and could well be the subject of a whole other book.

It is hoped that the political environment between the CEO and the medical staff is cooperative. When it is not, it is incumbent on the CEO to have an extraordinary amount of political savvy. As mentioned above, the CEO must evaluate his or her political savvy every 12 to 18 months. Experts have defined physicians and organized medical staffs as herd animals. A CEO who cannot penetrate the political motivation of a difficult medical staff would be doing himself or herself and the organization a great service by recognizing this and relocating to an organization where he or she could make better use of his or her administrative talent. A CEO who has the political finesse and savvy outlined above and who has sustaining power as evidenced by an ability to hold every level of the organization accountable for progress removes the focus of blame from the individual at the top (the CEO). In turn, all positive rewards can also be shared and enjoyed by all levels of the organization.

If there are some failures or setbacks, I cannot emphasize enough that nothing can be accomplished by attempting to put the blame on a weaker party. Whether one is dealing with the board, the medical staff, or employees, the sign of a good boss is one who takes more than his or her share of the blame and less than his or her share of the credit. However, when the CEO has outlined a series of problems that serve as the basis of the operational planning objectives for turning bad situations into win-win-win situations, as long as the medical staff is a part of those solutions and commits its own planning efforts to those of the administration and board, the CEO need not feel blameworthy or be publicly ostracized in a difficult political arena. For an abbreviated discussion on how to swim with sharks without bleeding or becoming a victim, I would refer you to the section below entitled Disemployment. In essence, the same axioms that pertain to an alternative for firing employees can easily and safely be applied to strained medical staff-CEO relationships. In brief, do not take possession of someone else's problem(s); to do so is to be held accountable for the solutions. Remember, as stated in step 5 of the planning process, I have never known a CEO to get into trouble when he or she maintained integrity, honesty, and passion for the organization.

Evaluations

A lot of articles and mandates, including those of the JCAHO, the American Hospital Association, and others, indicate that boards should be evaluated annually. However, I suspect that few boards in fact are. As a consequence, it might be perfectly appropriate for the CEO to assist the board in analyzing its accountability and effectiveness with a written summary of what they jointly accomplished in the year. This summary should include a review of how well it adhered to the operational planning objectives and, on a more critical note, a highlighting of the items the board did not support and the probable impact that resulted.

The performance of the medical staff must be evaluated against only the stated and agreed on objectives. Once the medical staff has assisted the CEO and the associate director or vice-president for clinical services in setting objectives for the medical staff that tie in with those stated by the board and administration, they too must be held accountable. With all due respect, the medical staff invariably needs administrative support to assist them in carrying through with institutional and clinical progress. Additionally, one could cite many examples of conflicts between the CEO and the medical staff on issues and policies that seemed to be legitimately established, but when a new medical staff leadership gets elected, their hierarchical memories become hazy at best. Almost annually, they begin to wonder why the hospital is operating according to a certain set of standards or requirements. It is helpful to be able to fall back on and retrace the operational planning that the medical staff has evaluated and supported over the years. Of course, not all decisions are intended to be set in concrete. But being able to defend how the institution arrived at a certain policy is extremely helpful in swimming in infested waters.

With respect to key managerial personnel, it is much easier to make the tough-call decisions with a system in place. Again, I refer the reader to the subsequent section regarding disemployment. If the department managers know that their objectives will be used as a basis of accountability and evaluation, they have a built-in incentive to perform to the maximum.

There is no harm or tragedy in deleting or deferring an operational objective as long as the manager can demonstrate an earnest attempt to implementing those goals. The underlying premise, again, is that once departmental managers have accepted responsibility for their territory, they have also agreed to be held accountable for their performance.

One remaining point is in order with respect to the evaluation of key managers. The best system of all is one that ties salary adjustments for managers to performance. The budget should set a percentage range that will be used as an incentive reward for outstanding performance, as an alternative to automatic cost-of-living or inflationary approaches. Salary adjustments should not be automatic.

Finally, the following elements should be commented on in narrative form in all key managerial evaluations: leadership, planning, organization, interaction (internal and external), control, judgment, and any general observations that can provide additional constructive input for enhancing motivation, performance, and productivity (Exhibit 5.4).

Retreats and Education

As stated above, by and large, the board of trustees and members of the medical staff who are fulfilling critical medico-administrative positions are volunteers. Time off from seeing patients or running other business interests costs these talented individuals time (leisure and family) and money. This cost might or might not be less important to some board members or medical staff leaders whose businesses or careers are very stable, but it is important to cultivate new and younger talent within the organization to prevent it from becoming static.

In approaching the educational needs of the board and medical staff leadership, board management and medical staff retreats can be extremely valuable in carrying out the finesse, politics, and planning objectives necessary for a multimillion dollar business to move forward in an increasingly competitive market. However, retreats must not only be of value to them personally but also be pertinent to their roles. It is a common mistake to bring in key speakers and set a retreat agenda that devotes too much time to what the administration or departmental managers need to be doing day to day to run the organization. Be cautious not to fall into the mistake of devoting one or two days to ingratiating the managerial efforts to them. One of two things will occur: either they will fall asleep, or they will redirect their support in ways that begin to challenge the CEO's day to day needs and decisions. The key, therefore, is to focus retreat topics

Exhibit 5.4 Criteria for Performance Evaluations

Factor	Criteria
Leadership	Ability to motivate others and also perhaps intitative, drive for excellence, special job knowledge, maintanance of high standards, and willingness to accept responsibility
Planning	Ability to develop worthwhile goals, design appropriate programs, and establish and maintain necessary budgets and timetables
Organization	Use of available resources to implement plans, the delegation of responsibility, and the assignment of specific duties
Interaction (internal)	Ability to work with others at the hospital to obtain and provide information and advice and to solve mutual problems
Interaction (external)	Ability to work with customers and other organizations to provide prompt and efficient service
Control	Ability to control costs and monitor programs and activities and adherence to plans, policies, and procedures
Judgment	Decision making, the establishment of priorities, the assessment of cost-benefit relationships, and willingness to make decisions

on their responsibilities and how they can become more productive within the organization. In so doing, the CEO's job becomes much more spontaneous and gratifying as the medical staff and board work on issues that are critical to the overall success of the organization while the CEO works on fine tuning the efficiency of the institution in a time of dwindling assets.

An example of acceptable retreat topics include issues relating to the medical-legal environment or reimbursement issues for the medical staff or joint venturing and new business opportunities or the management of the organization for the board. Avoid topics relating to the organizational structure needed to enhance your programs.

Regardless of the retreat topic selected, the real value of having retreats is to build consensus on the board objectives and to provide the entire organization with the green lights necessary to balance the organizational components that will enhance its diversified business programs. In essence, the process empowers the organization to go forward. Additionally, assuming that it has accepted and endorsed the CEO's strategic plan on each new business opportunity identified, the CEO has already answered questions of reimbursement and day-to-day management to its satisfaction. Once the CEO has the board's support in concept and its directions in establishing policy, the implementation phases become the sole prerogative of the CEO and the organization that exists to carry it out.

Whatever you do with respect to board management and medical staff leadership retreats, never make them feel stupid about the organization or insult their intelligence regarding what it will take for survival. Do not become so overzealous or enthused that they become uncomfortable with their own role or competence vis-à-vis their own organization or management style.

A brief note on trustee orientations: Frequently, the same trustees that motivated decisions five or ten years ago are moving on decisions that are of current importance. Unless they too have come along with the changes in the environment, they will cling to past traditions of decision making and prioritization. The CEO must regularly reorient the board from the traditional trustee role (long dead) to the new role of directorship. Here too there is a way to finesse the board into being excited about its own ability to think constructively in the best interests of the organization and into feeling positive about itself in committing its time and energy. The reader might recall that the sign of a good boss is one who takes less than his or her share of the credit, and I see no reason why the CEO should not give credit above in addition to below.

An annual or biennial trustees orientation should include as many trustees as possible to keep them current. The CEO should also have input into the chairperson's responsibility, committee assignments, and the determination of committee chairpeople and officers. The committee structure of a board is of paramount importance to its performance and productivity. To keep the board stimulated and productive, the chairperson's responsibilities should rotate. It takes years to achieve this development of the board, but, from my experience, everyone benefits in the end.

Disemployment

As I learned a long time ago, there are many ways to succeed yet one certain way to fail: by trying to please everyone. No CEO can resolve every problem and every organizational concern. However, it is incumbent on the CEO to facilitate decision making and problem solving. One way to succeed is to never take possession of another individual's problem. When it comes time to decide to remove an individual from an organization, it is not necessary to dehumanize the person in the process. Additionally, it is not at all necessary to be abrupt unless the person is being disemployed for cause. Parenthetically, when it is necessary to act abruptly and for cause, I too would agree with the terminology of *firing*. Short of that situation, an administrator can process out or disemploy an individual who is not producing to the level of the organization's need by taking a little extra time to *out process* them. The formula is fairly straightforward.

If, after a certain period of time, the CEO or an associate identifies a departmental manager, supervisor, or anyone else within the organization whose performance and productivity are not meeting agreed on standards and expectations, the person should be helped to identify the root of his or her problems. Once the administrator has summarized the problems that have resulted in the employee's failure to accomplish or achieve, the administrator should document them and present them to the employee to get him or her to agree with the administrator's assessment. Once the administrator has gotten the individual to agree that he or she has a problem or a set of problems, the administrator has taken the most important step in removing himself or herself from responsibility and accountability for the success or turnaround of the employee. The administrator must then get the employee to commit his or her solutions for how to turn his or her performance around to writing within a week or two. As a note of caution, the administrator should not embarrass the individual by requiring the written plan of correction to be typed by a secretary or office assistant. To do so is to invite rumors.

Assuming the individual is earnestly attempting to resolve his or her problems, he or she adheres to the agreed on timetable and offers the written plan of correction to the administrator. It is very important that the administrator be careful not to agree to a solution that the individual has attempted but failed at in the past—particularly if the solution previously originated through the administrator or with his or her assistance. This point is critical in disemploying another human being. The employee with a problem has a natural tendency to look up to his or her supervisor for advice and guidance. For the administrator to offer solutions to correct the problem completely aborts the entire process. An administrator who agrees on a course of action and a timetable for a solution that was directed by the administrator has only himself or herself to blame, if at the time of evaluation, the employee has failed.

On the other hand, if the individual, trying to excel and work within the organization, agrees that the identified problems are impairing his or her peak performance and the administrator agrees to the individual's written plan of correction (perhaps modified through discussion), one of two things happens:

1. The desired result would be that the individual will improve, address all the problem behavior, and ultimately become one of the best and most productive employees the administrator would ever hope to have on the organization's team.

2. The employee might recognize his or her inability to offer continued support and assistance to that particular institution. With the administrator's assistance, the employee can then conclude that he or she should take his or her talents to an organization where they can be maximized.

Few individuals should begin and end a career with one organization. Somehow the Japanese philosophy of indenturing their work force does not quite fit into our western culture. No matter what the issue, be it a superior-subordinate relationship, politics, or a major crisis that befalls the office or the organization, the administrator should not take possession of another individual's problems. The CEO should only take possession of and full responsibility for his or her own problems or those that the CEO has created. By maintaining his or her own integrity, the CEO can allow those with problems to maintain theirs. Any administrator who is intent on firing should consider all the emotional trauma and uncertainty that can destroy an individual's self-worth and esteem. One would be hardpressed to identify any circumstances in which it is to anyone's personal or the organization's benefit to destroy a human in addition to outprocessing them.

In Summary

Guiding the Organization from Confusion to Consensus

To turn the situation from one of chaos to collaboration, various strategic, structural, leadership, and management talents are crucial for success. Perhapssome of the most well respected experts in the behavioral sciences are Steven M. Shortell and Raymond F. Mickus. These experts have written a number of valuable articles that have touched the heart of organizational and managerial solvency. Perhaps one of the best articles I have ever seen them produce was published in the January/February 1986 issue of *Healthcare Forum*, entitled "Standing Firm on Shaky Ground."[1] In brief, their outline mirrors the strategy that DeGraff has followed over the past six years. The secret is not all that mysterious. The principles of this strategy are outlined in Exhibit 5.5.

The idea behind the outline in Exhibit 5.5 is to marry the eight underlying principles outlined in *In Search of Excellence* by Peters and Waterman[2] (Exhibit 5.6) and the dissection of managerial thought outlined in Harold Geneen's book, *Managing* (Exhibit 5.7), with one's own drive, passion, thoroughness, and thirst for results. The result is organization that treats quality assurance as a mandate and achieves it everyday. It is a little ironic that the JCAHO has struggled for years to set standards for quality. It mandates ongoing quality assurance activities throughout the institution and reporting to the board as a condition of monitoring the clinical programs offered within an institution. From an industry standpoint, it is embarrassing to think that the JCAHO has had to mandate quality assurance activities in our institutions. DeGraff (from my perspective) set the example.

I would like to make one final comment on the subject of quality assurance. Presumably, every CEO in the country and his or her board has committed to having a quality assurance coordinator or some tangible method for assuring that the quality of care continues to be monitored. Simply stated, if the board, administration, and medical staff target quality assurance as an operational objective for each business planning year, it follows that every department where quality can be measured also commits to the same objective. In essence, programs such as generic screening, ongoing reporting of variances, and other quality assurance programs become organizational second nature.

DeGraff now spends more time at each board meeting discussing quality than any other topic. Its monthly operational reports to the board regarding quality assurance activities are as formalized as its financial performance reports.

Results and Epilogue

Although functioning as a community hospital in New York State entails some tumultuous challenges, the board, management, and medical Staff would agree that DeGraff has turned the corner from a bleak outlook to one of strength, perseverance and prosperity. DeGraff Memorial Hospital's bright future must be credited to the collective commitment and sweat of

Exhibit 5.5   Principles for Guiding an Organization from Confusion to Consensus

---

Guidelines for Strategy

1. Develop collaborative arrangements with organizations different from yours.
2. Have a series of new services and markets continuously under development.
3. Discover and develop new market niches.
4. Consider alternatives to divestment of needed services.
5. Seek out opportunities to divest services.
6. Intensify efforts to price competitively and increase volume.
7. Know your competitors.
8. Cultivate "good competitors."

Guidelines for Making Structural Changes

1. Keep things small.
2. Keep things flexible.

Guidelines for Leadership and People Management

1. Raise your level of sensitivity to meanings and symbols.
2. Convert ambiguity, uncertainty and conflict into focused positive energy.
3. Take prudent risks.
4. Search for bold, robust decisions.

Source: S. M. Shortell and R. F. Mickus, "Standing Firm on Shaky Ground," *Healthcare Forum*, January/February 1986.

the board, medical staff, employees, and community at large. All concerned are indeed excited about its prospects.

Although the financial performance of hospitals in New York State cannot be equitably evaluated against those in the other 49 states, certain key indicators attest that DeGraff has indeed managed to turn around. The indicators are summarized below.

Management Structure

Over the past seven years, DeGraff has vertically integrated its corporate and management structure to include the establishment of the DeGraff

Exhibit 5.6 Lessons from America's Best-Run Companies

1. Maintain a bias for action (i.e., be willing to move, make decisions, and take risks).
2. Stay close to the customer (i.e., keep an open ear to your customers needs, wants, and expectations; satisfy their needs and anticipate their wants).
3. Maintain autonomy and entrepreneurship (i.e., be innovative and unique).
4. Increase productivity through people (i.e., trust your staff and they will produce).
5. Be hands on and value driven (i.e., set an organizational climate and corporate culture).
6. Stick to the knitting (i.e., do what you do best).
7. Have a simple form and lean staff (i.e., keep your organizational structure and your top management clean and streamlined; rely on your producers).
8. Incorporate simultaneous loose-tight properties (i.e., treat people decently and ask them to shine; produce things that work).

Source: T. J. Peters and R. H. Waterman, Jr., *In Search of Excellence* (New York: Harper & Row Publishers, 1982).

Holding Corporation, the DeGraff Memorial Hospital, the DeGraff Hospital Foundation, and DeGraff Enterprises, Inc. All four corporations are interrelated, with separate and distinct boards that represent a cross-section of the community. Managerially, DeGraff has vertically integrated to strengthen the core business on which it will flourish in the future. Included in this vertical integration is the enhancement of what was a 135-bed medical-surgical hospital into 185 beds with additional licensed and certified beds for acute rehabilitation and alternate level of care and an anticipated expansion of the long-term care beds in its skilled nursing facility with a second floor addition that will bring its total operating bed capacity to 265. This growth, expansion, and diversification is enhanced with new ambulatory programs such as 11 free-standing speech therapy clinics for all of Western New York and the only intergenerational day care program in Niagara County, which has 60 child care and 30 adult day care slots and a free-standing modern building. The hospital has purchased additional real estate on three separate sites for clinical office space in

Exhibit 5.7   Managing Tips

You cannot run a business, or anything else, on a theory.

Two Organizational Structures

Every company has two organizational structures: the formal one is written on the charts; the other is the everyday living relationship of the men and women in the organization.

Leadership

Leadership cannot really be taught. It can only be learned.

Disease

The worst disease that can afflict business executives in their work is not, as popularly supposed, alcoholism; it's egotism.

On Caring

The key element in good business management is emotional attitude.

Source: H. Geneen *Managing* (Garden City, New York: Doubleday & Company, Inc., 1984).

addition to a fourth building for an elder care program that provides outpatient and referral services to the elderly and their caregivers. Lastly, it has developed a business plan for occupational medicine that will put a high revenue producer into two distinct communities that are served within its corporate mission.

Community

Another test of the hospital's managerial turnaround has been the level of renewed support and enthusiasm by the majority of its community's citizens. The community is appreciative of the enhanced access to new primary care physicians, the services of our elder care program doing business as the McLaughlin Center, and increased diagnostic capabilities in virtually every outpatient departmental component including magnetic resonance imaging, computerized axial tomography (CAT) scanning, and a dedicated mammography program for women's health.

Medical Staff

In the view of the external medical community in Western New York, DeGraff has clearly gone from a hospital that was considered a benign or nonprovider of health care services in the 1960s and 1970s to one worthy of notice. The hospital has had to make some difficult decisions on medical staff discipline, but the result has been a measurable improvement in the quality of care and the peer review monitoring process. The State University of New York at Buffalo School of Medicine has also taken notice of the new focus for our medical staff recruitment and retention efforts and, in conjunction with a proposed merger plan, will be establishing DeGraff as a full university-affiliated hospital with medical teaching programs in family medicine.

Board of Directors

The willingness of both the board and the CEO to be accountable and set the appropriate focus and direction for DeGraff has given the board extraordinary strength and conviction in negotiating DeGraff's future from a position of strength rather than as a last-ditch effort to find a safe harbor. A testament to the board's commitment to quality and setting policy for the future is the JCAHO's recent award to DeGraff of an unconditional three-year accreditation. Perhaps more pertinent is the rigorous and often times nit-picking attitude of the New York State Department of Health through their comprehensive survey process. The commissioner of health's officers told the administration without any hesitation that DeGraff Memorial Hospital was the best hospital surveyed in all of Western New York since the comprehensive survey process was established two years ago. This accolade is perhaps the highest that the New York State Department could ever offer an institution, or its board, management, medical staff, and employees.

Merger

To conclude, DeGraff is presently actively negotiating to merge its four corporate entities with a large university (tertiary) medical center with two campuses (one in downtown Buffalo with 450 operating beds and a second hospital campus in the eastern suburbs with 150 operating beds). The proposal is for both institutions to bring an equal amount of emphasis, talent, and resources to the new relationship. According to the New York

State Department of Health, which is considering this arrangement, this is the first time two nondesperate institutions have sought the state health department's approval for a merger of corporations licensed through the public health laws of the State of New York. Although a lot of ground remains to be covered in the months ahead, it looks very favorable that these efforts will create the win-win-win situations that were outlined in the turnaround process listed as step 5 as well as develop the medical staff relationships that were discussed in this chapter.

Notes

1. S. M. Shortell and R. F. Mickus, "Standing Firm on Shaky Ground," *Healthcare Forum*, January/February 1986.
2. T. J. Peters and R. H. Waterman, Jr. *In Search of Excellence* (New York: Harper & Row Publishers, 1982).
3. H. Geneen, *Managing* (Garden City, NY: Doubleday & Co. Inc., 1984).

6

REVITALIZATION OF A RURAL HOSPITAL

Joseph M. Smith

Editors' Note: This chapter's uniqueness is that it describes what must be done if the hospital's staff is reduced to a level where the hospital cannot be operated with a further loss of employees but continues to operate at a significant financial loss. The role of the volunteers, employees at all levels, the medical staff, and the management team are described in some detail. The chapter should be particularly useful for all executives operating smaller health care institutions.

Overlooking the banks of the Cedar River, surrounded by lush green fields, stands Gladwin Area Hospital (GAH). To the casual observer, it is the typical rural facility built during the boom years of hospitals. A recently constructed long-term care facility also graces the campus. In 1960, financed by the Hill-Burton program and community donations, a 42-bed acute care hospital was built to replace an aging physician-owned structure. An energetic fund drive produced surprising results as this small farming community rallied to the cause of having its own community hospital. The early years were extremely successful. A high census prevailed, providing plentiful resources and excellent employment for the community. In the early 1970s an enthusiastic expansion program resulted in the construction of an inpatient substance abuse facility. Once again, Hill-Burton funds were used to finance the project. It opened in 1974, and it too was highly successful.

The community was pleased with the health care programs that were being offered. Physician practices thrived, and threats from the outside were essentially nonexistent.

By the late 1970s, change began to occur. Tired of long hours and the high risk of doing obstetrics, family practice physicians reduced or completely eliminated that area from their practices. Management made no effort to recruit an obstetrical specialist to fill the gap. Patients began to migrate to nearby Midland for obstetrical care. Once accustomed to traveling the 35 miles, they began to seek other specialty care at the larger, more progressive Midland Hospital Center. Faced with fewer than 180 births per year, high costs, and a predominantly Medicaid population, the board decided to close the obstetrics department, sending a shock wave through the community and signaling that GAH might be in trouble.

The substance abuse program experienced early success, but building code and program deficiencies caused the state to force the closure of the entire program. The almost new building with substantial debt stood empty and began draining the increasingly scarce resources of the hospital. In an effort to salvage what was left, management converted the structure into physician offices. Rental rates below market value were offered to physicians while the hospital subsidized the difference, resulting in substantial ongoing losses.

Inpatient activity was declining steadily. The loss of obstetrics services and an eroding market share for general medical and surgical services began taking its toll on the profitability of the organization. The medical staff was aging and becoming increasingly conservative. The only general surgeon on the staff dramatically reduced his surgical practice and converted it to a general practice.

While all other hospitals were preparing themselves for the advent of the prospective payment system (PPS), management at GAH could not provide the leadership to redirect the thinking of the medical staff. Practice patterns remained unchanged while losses under the new reimbursement program steadily mounted. Excessive lengths of stay, coupled with unnecessary admissions, caused the Health Care Finance Administration to issue a warning that the hospital's provider status was in jeopardy. Reserves were quickly depleted and failure appeared imminent. In 1984, the board realized that the debt-burdened organization was in serious trouble and began formal affiliation negotiations with MidMichigan Regional Health System, which is the parent company of Midland Hospital Center, now known as MidMichigan Regional Medical Center. The formal agreement, signed in 1985, marked the beginning of a new era for the hospital and for the community. The year following the affiliation was filled with difficult decisions, major capital investments, and intensive repositioning. GAH now enjoys a more stable financial outlook and is once again significantly contributing to the health care delivery system of the mid-Michigan area. Although inpatient occupancy still hovers around 50 percent, GAH enjoys a better census than many small hospitals in the region. Outpatient business is brisk as the result of a repositioned emergency room and a new walk-in care program. Radiology services were enhanced by the addition of mobile CAT scanning. Ultrasound and a state-of-the-art Women's Breast Screening Program are offered in pleasant surroundings.

A comprehensive community health education program offers a wide array of educational programs for all age groups. The education center occupies an area once cluttered with old furniture and obsolete files.

The converted substance facility is fully occupied by staff physicians and visiting specialists from MidMichigan Regional Medical Center. Rental rates are competitive with area professional buildings, and the revenue covers the debt service and overhead. As the hospital's reputation improved, it once again became attractive to new physicians. The developing relationship with a larger hospital provided recruiting incentives for doctors who were once reluctant to practice in an isolated medical community. For these reasons, recruitment efforts led to the addition of a general surgeon, an internist, and three general practice physicians.

The hospital's financial performance is significantly improved. Following years of operating losses around $250,000 per year, income from operations is close to breaking even. In the first year following affiliation, subsidies from the parent company of $50,000 per month were necessary to maintain cash flow and to fund survival strategies. Without investing in the hospital, its demise would have been swift, leaving a vacuum in the health care system of the area. Subsidies are no longer required, and some of the initial cash infusion has been repaid.

Recognizing the importance of long-term care for the survival of this facility, a decision was made to redirect resources into building a nursing home. The Gladwin market was ripe for the development of a high quality skilled nursing facility. Through aggressive leadership and with the financial backing of the parent company, a 120-bed facility was constructed on the campus. Although it is independent of the hospital, it is attached to it and shares support services such as dietary, maintenance, pharmacy, and physical therapy. The facility opened in the fall of 1988, creating almost 100 new jobs and signaling the rebirth of the local health care program.

Understanding the Situation

The complex organizational problems at GAH were compounded by the inertia of a tradition-bound management group. The board, although appropriately motivated to effect change, could not relight the fires of the organization without dramatic management reorganization. To create a better environment for change, the CEO was replaced and several members of the management team voluntarily resigned or were reassigned.

The task of the new management team was clear. The financial hemorrhage had to be controlled. Before any additional resources were infused, the potential of the organization had to be assessed. Although the market was important to the parent corporation because of its location and the referrals for secondary and tertiary care, the cost of maintaining that market appeared excessive.

Long-range planning was almost impossible because the situation changed daily. Consequently, management chose to focus on the establishment and accomplishment of critical short-term objectives while formulating broad long-range strategic options. The short term objectives were

1. to assess operations, identify cost-reduction opportunities, and implement those that achieved a fast return on investment;
2. to evaluate staffing needs and human resource availability and adjust staffing to respond quickly to fluctuations in volume;
3. to analyze community perceptions and initiate effective communication designed to reestablish credibility;
4. to inventory the skills of the medical staff, identify barriers to effective practice under DRGs, and correct overutilization problems;
5. to ascertain the extent of financial liability and outline financial options; and
6. to identify the high-cost/low-return programs to determine if any should be divested to eliminate system duplication.

Operations Assessment

Cost-reduction opportunities are present in every organization. Identifying and implementing the steps for achieving results takes an organizationwide effort. For this project, GAH used the Operations Improvement Survey methodology developed at the MidMichigan Regional Medical Center. Each department manager completed the comprehensive survey. It assessed service delivery, customer satisfaction, supply consumption, staffing utilization, market potential, progress effectiveness, and intradepartmental systems. From the information, the administration formulated a list of operations improvement objectives and distributed them to the appropriate departments for completion. Of the 78 objectives developed from the survey, 95 percent were completed within the first year.

For example, through the operations improvement survey process, the administration identified a number of staff reduction opportunities. It became apparent that the organization was not effectively adjusting staff to account for day-to-day volume fluctuations. Staffing patterns were designed to respond to peaks in activity rather than the average. Through a series of staff reduction programs including layoffs, reassignments, and shortened hours, the adjusted FTEs per occupied bed were reduced from 4.15 to 3.65. The target of 3.15 was not achievable because of fixed staffing requirements in a few departments that made further reductions inappropriate.

The administration had poor information about the consumer's perception of the hospital. It needed to know if the community valued the hospital and was interested in utilizing its services. A community survey, randomly mailed throughout the service area, showed an interesting pattern. Overwhelmingly, the public expressed dissatisfaction with the availability and quality of physicians, the price of services, the quality of the facility, and the attitude of the hospital's staff. GAH clearly had an image problem that the hospital staff and its physicians perpetuated. In essence, the organization was its own worst enemy. Another survey finding showed that the public wanted the hospital in the community for two major reasons: to have 24-hour emergency room services available and to provide jobs in the community.

From the survey, it became apparent that the hospital had to do the following:

- Recruit physicians acceptable to more of the patient population.
- Focus on quality improvement and appropriate pricing in the emergency room.
- Improve the appearance of the facility.
- Improve the customer relations skills of physicians and employees.
- Establish the hospital as a quality employer and a good business neighbor.

Medical Staff Needs

Gladwin Area Hospital was a battle zone in the area of physician relations. Under the prior administration, there were no lines of communication between management and the medical staff. The board received either filtered medical staff information from the administration or complaints directly from the staff. Hostility, distrust, and outright efforts to derail new programs were prevalent.

Immediate steps to reverse these attitudes were critical to the revitalization program. By using the results of the consumer survey, we were able to convince key physicians that the lack of depth in the medical staff was a serious problem. Recruitment of additional practitioners was critical to the hospital's future. The concept was not enthusiastically endorsed, but at least there were no overt efforts to make it fail. New physicians were gradually accepted.

Financial Analysis

While most organizations wrestle with the formulation of long-term financial plans, GAH was struggling to meet day-to-day cash requirements. The hospital was living from payday to payday and ignoring the requests of its suppliers for payment of past due accounts. Accounts receivable were increasing, and collection efforts were minimal. Cash flow was further threatened by demands from the third-party payers to repay overpayments from the interim payment programs. With no debt capacity available, it became necessary to seek subsidies from the parent company in the form of supplies and services. A projection showed that if financial operations were not controlled, the subsidy would exceed $1 million within two years.

A five-year financial forecast based on current activity and expenditure levels showed that losses would continue to increase. Management explored bankruptcy as an option. It was rejected because the hospital would never recover. Instead, a financial performance improvement plan was developed with the following objectives:

- Reduce labor costs to the absolute minimum.
- Authorize only critical expenditures.
- Aggressively collect outstanding accounts.
- Invest in new revenue generating programs.
- Eliminate the subsidization of physician offices.

Program Divestiture

Traditional cost-reduction efforts do not always produce results rapidly enough to reverse serious financial losses. It is sometimes necessary to cut off a service or program that has high costs and no financial return. When

GAH analyzed its programs, it became apparent that any divestiture would result in unacceptable levels of patient care. Obstetrical services had already been eliminated with damaging results. Although eliminating surgery was targeted as a possible cost-reduction measure, studies showed that low volume was the result of inadequate surgeon coverage rather than a weak market. Instead of divesting this program and others, management decided to invest in them by improving the quality and availability. A surgeon was recruited to boost surgical volume. Equipment was added to radiology to enhance imaging capability and retain patients that would otherwise be transferred. Laboratory equipment was upgraded to improve turnaround time. The emergency room was reorganized to include an effective urgent care program.

Key Players

The financial and operational problems facing GAH were enormous, and time was rapidly running out. Opportunities to fundamentally change the direction of the organization existed but seemed beyond the grasp of the organization. Some hoped that the affiliation with MidMichigan Regional Health Systems would magically solve all the hospital's problems. Unfortunately, the affiliation was only a first step in the process. The real work of changing the organization for the better and eventually improving its performance began after the affiliation was completed. Each member of the organization would be called on to demonstrate personal commitment to the process and to contribute to the achievement of established objectives. In the turnaround at GAH, several groups played critical roles. Some were the driving force behind success, while others drained the energy of the organization, making the turnaround more difficult to achieve.

The Board

Small community hospital boards are often made up of the best and the brightest from business, industry, and the public sector. GAH's board was typical in its composition. Each member was well known in the community and was held responsible for the success or the failure of the hospital. The threat of complete closure weighed heavily on the board, and it collectively decided to do everything possible to avoid failure.

The board room became the equivalent of a war room during a major battle. Strategy formulation, position assessments, the evaluation of options, and damage control were frequent discussion subjects. As management refined the assessment of the hospital's operations and communicated it to the board, it became apparent that tough decisions were necessary. Layoffs, wage reductions, and other painful cost-reduction measures filled the agenda of meetings. The board tried to minimize individual employee hardship yet meet financial targets. Local economic impact was weighed with each decision. Decisions that served only the hospital's interests at the expense of the community were modified to benefit both.

Personal commitment from individual board members was essential in the revitalization process. During the most difficult period, meetings were held almost daily so that vital decisions were not delayed. This board had to act decisively and collectively. Once a difficult decision was reached, each member worked with his or her constituencies in the community to help them understand why the decision was made and how it would affect them. This communication became a powerful public relations tool that eased the organization through a difficult transition.

No one expected to have a simple job as a hospital trustee. GAH's situation tested the board to a great degree. Many weaker governing bodies would have bailed out of this situation rather than face the fears, struggles, and potential failure. Rather than relaxing once the crisis was over, this board maintained the same intensity and channeled it into future developments.

Management Team

Hospitals that encounter serious financial and operating deficiencies are frequently undermanaged. GAH's management problems had to be corrected before undertaking the turnaround effort. A lack of leadership and financial ineptitude were the two underlying deficiencies. Medical staff shortages and regulatory pressures were rapidly eroding the financial base. Nursing floundered because qualified staff could not be recruited. Within less than six months, three new administrators were hired. The new team, although relatively inexperienced, applied sound management techniques that began to show results within the year.

Changes were also made in the structure of the organization below the senior management level. Some department head positions were combined, and several supervisory positions were eliminated. The administration found a tremendous pool of enthusiasm in the supervisory group that had previously been untapped. Because of senior management's commitment to a participative style, supervisors developed ownership in the turnaround process and became an important catalyst for effective change. Each accomplishment was hailed as forward progress. The success experienced by managers created enthusiasm that was contagious. Additional responsibilities were assigned to lower level supervisors who showed significant management potential. This strategy allowed the organization to accomplish many projects without the addition of management staff.

Medical Staff

A successful turnaround project is difficult under ideal circumstances. When the medical staff does not cooperate, the process is complicated further. At GAH, physicians were entrenched in the traditional role of an adversary with administration. Each management decision was viewed with suspicion. When a physician did cooperate with management, he was accused of breaching the solidarity of the entire staff. With a change in top management, a small window of opportunity to cooperate opened. As a group, the staff hung tenaciously to traditional ideas, yet they could be individually convinced that change was necessary and that new ideas would eventually work to their advantage. It quickly became apparent that this group of doctors reacted negatively to change because of the fear of lost revenue and the loss of autonomy. Management had no choice but to clearly demonstrate to them that in many instances they were the direct cause of the hospital's financial problems. They could no longer ignore the DRG System, and they had to become more responsive to the patients of the community.

The CEO made several attempts to show them that the hospital could not survive without their help and that they could not continue to practice effectively without the hospital. Once they were convinced that the hospital's success was closely tied to their own economic future, cooperation was more frequent. Gradually, a few came to the conclusion that additional doctors were pivotal if the hospital was to succeed. The most conservative physicians never embraced the concept, but fortunately, reason prevailed. As new doctors came on board, the balance of power began to shift to those who were more progressive, and the medical staff began to work in cooperation with the hospital.

Management worked hard to earn the trust of the doctors through frequent sharing of ideas, keeping them informed, and providing them with solutions for their problems. Although the relationship was never perfect, it improved enough to allow progress to occur.

Employees

Gladwin Area Hospital is the second largest employer in the county. Historically, the hospital was viewed as the ideal place to work because of high pay and secure jobs. Favoritism and nepotism were common employment practices. The community viewed the hospital as a closed system with only the privileged few allowed to apply for jobs. With a limited pool of employees, negative attitudes among groups were self-perpetuating. Except for management and clerical workers, all employees were represented by the United Steel Workers of America. Shortly after the affiliation, fearing the loss of their own jobs, the clerical workers joined forces with the other employees and voted to be represented.

The local union had a long history of intimidating management into expensive compensation programs and unrealistic job security provisions. In the environment of the 1980s, these programs only exacerbated the financial situation. The analysis of the work force clearly showed that the hospital was overstaffed and inefficient. A layoff of almost 40 employees could not be avoided and was implemented. The layoff hardened the union's position with contract negotiations less than a year away.

Employee morale was at an all-time low. Although the layoffs were completed, the remaining employees feared that more reductions were inevitable. Patients sensed the employee dissatisfaction and were reluctant to be hospitalized at GAH, causing further volume decreases.

Management employed a dual strategy in dealing with this problem. It stepped up the communication to all levels through a series of employee meetings held around the clock. The facts about the hospital's condition were shared with everyone, dispelling rumors and half truths. Management then informed the union that it needed to open labor talks early to reach an agreement that could help the hospital survive. It informed the union that a labor cost-reduction was absolutely necessary to reduce the growing deficit.

When management unveiled its wage and benefit concession package, the union leadership convinced its membership that the hospital was better off than they were led to believe. Talks continued with little progress for two months, and the expiration of the contract was fast approaching. The threat of a strike became apparent. Management was convinced that it could not safely operate the hospital through a labor dispute and developed a simple strike plan: Transfer all patients to other facilities, close the acute care hospital, and operate the emergency room with management personnel.

Management made no secret of the plan, and it quickly became common knowledge. The holding company agreed that this course of action would eventually result in permanent closure of the acute care facility with the possibility of only an outpatient center remaining. After weighing the odds of financial failure if concessions were not granted against the negative effects of a strike, management privately agreed to risk a strike and proceed with permanent closure if a strike occurred.

Fortunately, with the assistance of a federal mediator, a concession contract yielding 16.5 percent in wage reductions was finally ratified without a labor dispute. The end of the negotiations signaled the turning point. Employees realized that they must now be active participants in the process of change if success was to be achieved. Because of management's honest and straightforward approach, attitude and morale improved, and the hospital began to function once again. Employees began contributing to new programs by volunteering their time and talents to new projects. The new contract provided avenues for professional growth through tuition reimbursement and rewards for exceptional performance through a bonus system. When the hospital generated a surplus in the year following the wage reductions, over $50,000 in performance bonuses were distributed to employees.

Volunteers

The spirit of volunteers was one of the brightest aspects of GAH. The hospital auxiliary had more than 100 members who were ready and willing to take up the challenge of making the hospital succeed. The auxiliary president was an enthusiastic woman with boundless energy and dedication. Her executive committee had become frustrated that its earlier efforts to establish new programs or make meaningful contributions had not been supported.

Sensing the value of this untapped resource, the new administration called the volunteers into action. They were designated as the primary public relations force. They carried the hospital's message to the community regularly. Management shared its ideas with them, and they provided valuable input into its decisions. Some administrators view their volunteer group only as an alternative source of revenue because their donations fund many important projects. At GAH, the volunteers had historically provided only small contributions because they were not encouraged to do otherwise. They had a significant uncommitted reserve. Rather than soliciting funds from the auxiliary, management chose to enhance their image in the hospital and provide meaningful programs for them to manage. In a short time, volunteers were active in almost every department. They helped patients with menus, gave tours to the public, and assisted with diagnostic screening programs and many other projects. They were enthusiastically asking to do more. Eventually, their financial contributions became just as significant. Through their efforts, funds were raised to redecorate the entire hospital, a mobile CAT scan dock was built and dedicated to their honor, the patient tray service was modernized to provide attractive hot meals, and emergency room monitoring equipment was purchased. Each donation was received with high publicity in the papers and throughout the community. The motivating force behind the volunteers' efforts was appreciation for the work they do. GAH valued their personal donations of time as much as their financial contributions. The turnaround could not have succeeded without their exceptional efforts.

External Factors Affecting Revitalization

Government Programs

Not many hospital administrators view the PPS, peer review organizations (PROs), Health Care Finance Administration (HFCA), and the Hill-Burton program as positive forces for change. These programs had a significant influence on GAH and indirectly transformed the hospital from an inefficient resource-consuming machine into a vehicle for cost-effective health care delivery.

The advent of the PPS signaled the need for dramatic changes at the hospital. For years, inefficiencies compounded while the market slipped away. Under the PPS, the government refused to pay for waste and unnecessary care. GAH was forced to change its outdated operating methods or suffer irreparable financial damage. Doctors had to submit to the scrutiny of the PRO, which judged the care they provided. The HCFA refused to pay the hospital if care was inappropriate. Hill-Burton loans helped build the hospital but, as a condition, required the facility to provide ever-increasing amounts of free care. This care has to be delivered as economically as possible to balance the financial losses.

Without the influence of these programs in the early 1980s, GAH might never have realized that its position was dramatically eroding. While some administrators blame these programs for the decline of their hospitals, they fail to realize that their hospital was likely failing long before the programs were instituted. GAH was one of those hospitals. It was consuming itself by not reinvesting in its plant, by overpaying its employees for inefficient work, and by ignoring its responsibilities to the community. This hospital, like so many others, was taking itself for granted. It assumed it was insulated from financial problems because governmental programs ignored efficiency and rewarded waste. If government programs had remained as they were before DRGs, this hospital might initially have avoided the hardship it encountered, but it would probably have suddenly failed with no chance of revival.

Press and Media Relations

Throughout the revitalization, national media attention was focused on the plight of hospitals. Hospital failures made headlines in many cities. Mortality statistics were published, stripping away the historic immunity hospitals enjoyed. National attention to health care issues caused the local media to scrutinize the local hospital. GAH used the unusually high exposure to capitalize on opportunities to communicate its unique problems without sending negative messages. The administration managed the press by keeping them informed of the hospital's positive progress while providing them with advance notice of any potential negative measures it had to implement. Without blaming or complaining, it informed the press that those steps were necessary if the hospital was to survive this difficult period and plan for its future. Rather than issuing short press releases after the fact, management called in key members of the media before action was taken. It communicated its story and provided them with fact sheets. It was successful in keeping the public informed while minimizing the appearance of an insurmountable crisis. The results of management's efforts were great. Throughout the turnaround, not one negative news article was published except a letter to the editor from a dissatisfied employee.

Our public relations efforts also included frequent talks to civic groups, governmental bodies, and private clubs. Each time the message was the same: the hospital is struggling to survive, but it will emerge in a better position to serve the community's needs.

Effective press and public relations in a turnaround is vital for success. No group is quicker to criticize than an uninformed press. Newspaper articles that are carefully planned strengthen the hospital's image in the eyes of the most important audience—the patient.

The Holding Company

The turnaround of GAH may be unique. Even though the catalyst for change came from the affiliation with MidMichigan Regional Health System, the local hospital itself was required to provide the necessary leadership. The revitalization process was a joint effort between local leadership and the leadership of the system. Even though the holding company provided financial support, management expertise, and planning assistance when the hospital requested, the local board made the decision to implement the recommended changes. The parent company did not usurp the responsibilities of the local board or management, choosing instead to act as a consultant. This approach strengthened the relationship between the two organizations and created an environment where trust and security prevailed. Local decision makers remained in control of their own destiny and took responsibility for their decisions. This approach differs from that used by other health care systems, who often dictate all decisions from afar.

MidMichigan Regional Health System valued the market served by GAH. It represented an important referral source for its services. Additionally, MidMichigan Regional Health System had a long history of concern for the rural areas, and GAH was an important link in that market. Therefore, it invested heavily in the hospital and added a $4 million nursing home to the campus. The new facility improved access to long-term care in the county and demonstrated the system's commitment to that market. Allowing flexibility in local decision making and establishing a long-term commitment to the community are key components of a successful turnaround when a larger system is involved in the management of a rural hospital.

Remaining Challenges

Turnaround projects are usually described as having a beginning and a conclusion. Success is often declared when the income statement shows a positive bottom line. Unfortunately, small hospitals cannot stop there. The future will likely bring additional struggles that could once again plunge the organization into financial trouble. Competition, regulation, and technology will continue to reshape the health care industry, often at the expense of a small hospital's future.

The challenge that lies ahead for GAH is to continually assess its position in the market and anticipate the course corrections that will be necessary to address future challenges. Maintaining the status quo cannot become its operating objective. Throughout this chapter, it has been clear that the hospital's problems were linked to deficiencies in leadership. Without improving the skills of those in key positions or replacing them with others who could effectively lead the organization, the turnaround might not have been as successful. This hospital and others like it will have difficulty attracting and retaining true leaders to their boards and management teams. Small hospitals are a difficult arena in which to practice the art of successful management. They are neither a stepping stone for the inexperienced or a retirement haven for worn out managers.

The medical staff also played an important role in the turnaround process. Without continual replenishment of the staff and the expansion of its capabilities, the future of the hospital will be jeopardized. Successful physician recruitment will be expensive and frustrating. Attracting doctors who have a genuine commitment to the practice of rural medicine will be a critical success factor.

Postproject Analysis

After the smoke of the battle clears, the commander surveys the battlefield. Even though victorious, one asks oneself if one made the right decisions. Could casualties have been reduced? Could fewer vital resources have been consumed? Could the battle have been shortened? Turnaround projects are the equivalent of battle. There are casualties, and valuable resources are expended. Significant time commitments are necessary. While some turnaround efforts are successful, others fail in spite of valiant efforts. The GAH project was successful because of tremendous personal and organizational commitment. In retrospect, the results might have been achieved sooner, with fewer resources consumed, if a slightly different approach in the following areas were used.

Cost Reductions

Management chose to implement staff reductions gradually over a year. Throughout that year, employee morale suffered, and productivity was low. If the reductions had been swift and completed early in the process, financial losses would have been reduced, and the uncertainty experienced by employees would have been minimized. Management learned that after an affiliation or merger, all employees expect change. Management should carefully plan, clearly communicate, and swiftly implement the changes it must eventually make. Prolonging the process only frustrates the objectives.

Financial Support

In the early stages of this project, the holding company infused significant financial resources into GAH to maintain operations. This approach was chosen to minimize the risk of financial failure. In reality, it might have contributed to the perpetuation of organizational inefficiencies. I now feel that if a hospital lacks a ready source of money, it will be forced into financial independence much more rapidly and will make the necessary adjustments if it is motivated to survive. If subsidization is necessary, funds should be advanced only for programs that improve the organization's ability to attract and retain a critical mass of business. Subsidies advanced to cover operating shortfalls might delay the turnaround.

Medical Staff Development

The small medical staff at GAH vigorously protected its independence and demanded that autonomy be guaranteed after the affiliation. To expedite reaching an agreement, MidMichigan Regional Health Service agreed to that demand. The doctors were disfranchised during the affiliation negotiation and never owned the process or the outcome. The lesson learned was that doctors are a critical component of the turnaround, and they should have been brought into the process of the affiliation and turnaround early. Risk-sharing programs should have been implemented. This approach might have strengthened their resolve to cooperate and might have encouraged their active participation. Instead, they were permitted to act as casual observers who criticized important decisions and stalled the implementation of key programs.

Summary

A successful turnaround occurs when the leadership of the organization is motivated to create an effective environment for change. The following are key lessons that can be learned from the GAH's experience:

- Critically assess the organization; capitalize on the strengths and rapidly correct the weaknesses.

- The board of directors can effect change only if it is provided with information that identifies the problem and proposes solutions.
- The management team must function in concert with the board and have a clearly defined purpose.
- Communication to employees, the press, volunteers, and the community must be frequent, factual, and positive.
- Physicians must be encouraged to support the turnaround; otherwise, they will seriously impede progress.
- To improve financial results, cost reductions alone will not be effective; they must be coupled with market improvements.
- Difficult decisions must be made swiftly with full awareness of the personal and community input.
- The organization must focus on short-term improvements while simultaneously developing its long-term vision.
- Financial independence should be forced as soon as possible.
- Maintain the momentum of the turnaround process to avoid a prolonged struggle.

A turnaround project is never complete. Reversing negative financial results should not be the only goal of a turnaround. A positive bottom line is only the result of the achievement of many objectives. Periodic reassessment of the organization's position throughout the process leads to the establishment of additional objectives for future development. Relaxation of the spirit of enthusiasm and commitment that sparked a successful turnaround can lead to a reversal in a short time. Small rural hospitals can never relax and enjoy easy success. Many might be resuscitated time after time, but in the long run, many will have difficulty guaranteeing their future. GAH cannot guarantee its future either. However, from the lessons it learned, it will be better prepared to react when financial and operational pressures once again threaten its viability.

7

EXPENSE REDUCTIONS AND REVENUE INCREASES IN A HOSPITAL TURNAROUND

William D. Nicely and Joan E. Neuhaus

Editors' Note: This chapter highlights one of the most dramatic and sustained turnarounds in the United States. The health care corporation went from a net operating loss one year to a bottom line from operations of $4.6 million operating income the next year to $6.9 million the following year to over $8 million from operations the last year that is chronicled in the turnaround process. There is considerable focus not only on the expense portion of the equation but also on the revenue side. It is, in terms of the need for both expense reductions and revenue increases, one of the most balanced turn-arounds described in the book.

Like death and taxes, one more thing is certain today in health care: change. The health care industry has experienced major change in nearly every aspect of the business in the past ten years. And there is every indication that the 1990s promise to hold more of the same. The response of hospitals to this constant barrage of new development has been as varied as the hospitals themselves. Hospitals have tried everything from diversification to consolidation in their struggle to adapt and survive. Archbishop Bergan Mercy Hospital (ABMH) in Omaha, Nebraska, is no different from its counterparts in this respect. It has gone through a volatile marketplace adjustment and experienced a severe financial downturn. This chapter recounts some of the struggles and strategies that helped Bergan Mercy Hospital emerge a strong organization that is better equipped to anticipate and respond to the future.

The Situation

Archbishop Bergan Mercy Hospital is a 470-bed, acute care hospital and a 250-bed skilled nursing facility owned and operated by the Religious Sisters of Mercy. The hospital has a medical staff of over 500 and more than 2,000 employees. The Omaha health care marketplace, which includes the adjacent community of Council Bluffs, Iowa, is extremely competitive.

Eleven acute care hospitals (excluding military and veterans facilities) and two medical schools serve a population of roughly 600,000 people. Like most other areas of the country, inpatient utilization declined from 1984 to 1988 and is only now beginning to stabilize. Unlike some other parts of the country, however, the higher-than-average hospital usage in the eleven Omaha–Council Bluffs hospitals exacerbated the problem. When the shift to fixed reimbursement and the emphasis on outpatient treatment came, Omaha hospitals experienced a much larger drop in inpatient census because of a traditionally higher use rate than other areas of the country. So while the nation as a whole experienced, on the average, 3 percent annual reductions in acute inpatient admissions (defined as medical-surgical, obstetrics, and pediatric admissions), Omaha experienced a 10 percent annual reduction.[1,2] Acute patient days per 1,000 population (defined as medical-surgical, obstetrics, and pediatrics census days) fell from 1,115 per 1,000 in 1984 to 750 per 1,000 in 1988, a 32 percent drop.[3] Average acute occupancy for all Omaha hospitals dropped from 62.7 percent of licensed bed capacity (based on a total of 3,310 acute beds among 11 hospitals) in 1984 to 43.0 percent in 1988.[4] (See Figure 7.1.)

In addition to too many beds, two other factors influenced the downturn in the Omaha market. Nebraska has had a strong certificate-of-need law in effect, which placed significant barriers for hospitals to add new inpatient or outpatient services. As a result, the freedom to implement new hospital services was limited and the competition to increase or maintain existing patient volumes was intense. Managed care health plans, after a slow start, began to have real impact in 1986, introducing a whole new set of players to the market with an agenda to capture marketshare and to reduce reimbursement for all hospital services.

In 1985 and 1986 ABMH reacted like many other hospitals at that time—with a flurry of activity. The hospital merged with another hospital owned by the Sisters of Mercy in Council Bluffs and formed the parent company, Mercy Midlands. It added staff at the corporate level and began actively pursuing other merger candidates to extend its referral base into rural communities of Nebraska and Iowa. The number of corporations and

Figure 7.1 Percentage of Change in Inpatient Admissions: Omaha Area Versus Nationally

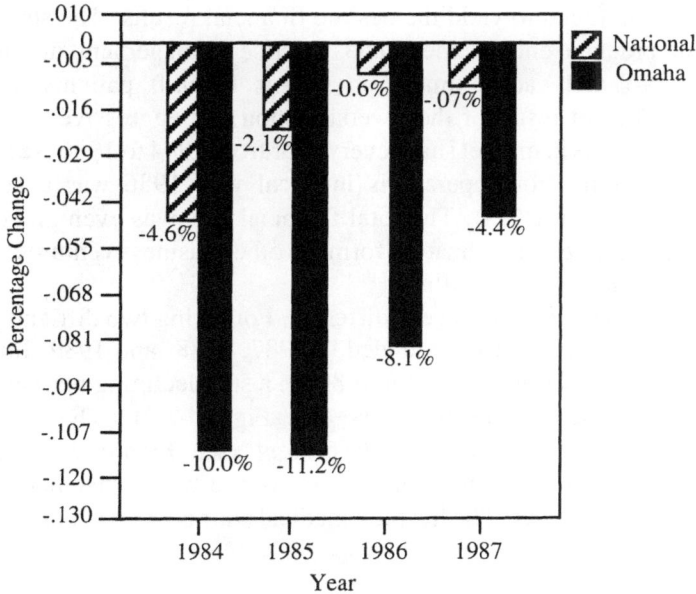

Sources: AHA, *Economic Trends;* State of Nebraska, Department of Health.

business ventures proliferated; the expenses and staff to support them also expanded. A for-profit entity was formed to handle joint ventures for the medical staff. Physician practices were purchased and other office practice enhancements were introduced. New lines of business, such as wellness and health promotion and a women's resource center were added. Retail pharmacies and durable medical equipment ventures were begun. Aggressive advertising campaigns were implemented with extensive television and print programs aimed at the public. The popular literature and the health care gurus of the time advocated becoming a comprehensive, integrated health care system with expanded revenue sources. With that advice in mind, but without a plan or specific business goals, Bergan Mercy pursued a multitude of ventures and new businesses.

In mid-1986, ABMH, the flagship of the system, was in trouble. Costs were soaring as a result of all the new ventures and activities at the same time that inpatient utilization was at an all-time low. Many of the new ventures, hurried into operation, had little planning and ill-defined profit objectives and failed to yield the desired financial results. The strategy of physician practice enhancement and practice management divided the medical staff and caused many physicians to shift patients to other hospitals. The net result of the diversification and aggressive expansion strategy was a loss in market share every year from 1984 to 1986 (see Figure 7.2). Net income from operations in fiscal year 1986 was a negative $188,000 (see Figure 7.3). The total financial loss was even greater due to losses in the parent organization form the other business ventures, which amounted to nearly $1.7 million.

In 1989 ABMH looked very different. Following two difficult years, market share and earnings rebounded in 1987, 1988, and 1989. Inpatient admissions increased in fiscal year 1989, in a still declining market place, the first such increase in six years (see Figure 7.2).[5] The hospital's operating margin increased to 9.6 percent (see Figure 7.3) and the hospital's image in the community, as measured by a consumer survey, has never been stronger. The hospital medical staff is more cohesive; it has

Figure 7.2   Archbishop Bergan Mercy Hospital Market Share

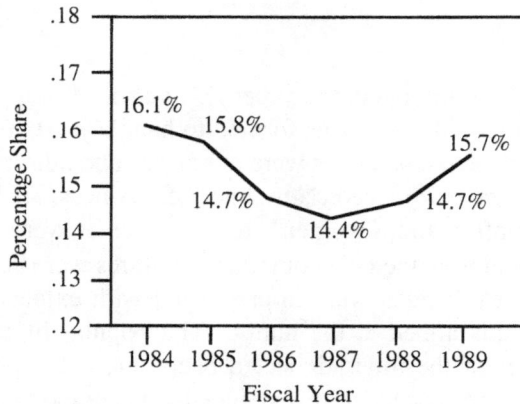

Source: State of Nebraska, Department of Health.

Figure 7.3 Archbishop Bergan Mercy Hospital Net Operating Revenue

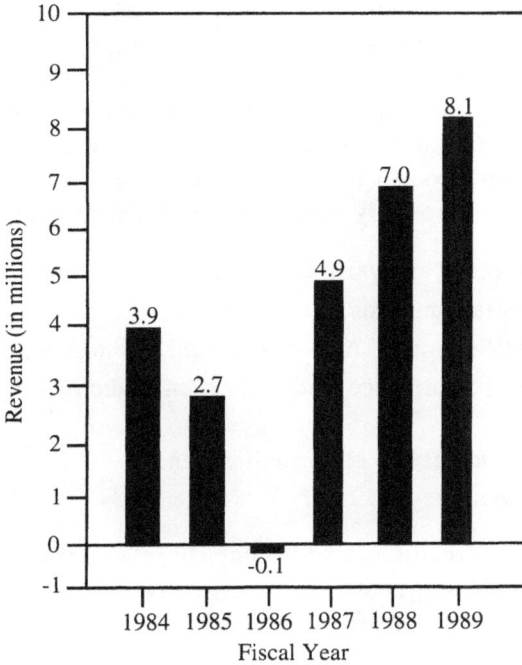

brought 29 new physicians to the staff, 7 of these recruited to fill specific specialties identified in the strategic planning process. ABMH has emerged stronger, leaner, more efficient, and ready to respond to the challenges ahead.

Diagnostics

The road back to health began in the fall of 1986 when the board of directors, faced with mounting losses, committed to a comprehensive strategic planning process. As part of that process, three immediate actions were taken:

1. A change in top management was made.
2. A moratorium was placed on new projects or ventures until a more comprehensive planning process was implemented.

3. One hundred twenty FTE positions were eliminated, to lower operating costs to be more in line with the reduction in patient census.

Strategic planning is one of the most difficult, most time-consuming, and least understood of the board and management functions. J. X. Reynolds and Co., Inc., management consultants, was retained to assist in the development of the strategic plan. Hospital procedures and services were grouped into product lines and the internal and external operation environment was thoroughly analyzed. The finished plan included

- a marketplace analysis,
- medical staff analysis,
- the identification of ABMH strategic business units,
- financial performance and utilization objectives for all business units,
- product and service opportunities, and
- goals and strategies.

Armed with the information gained through the planning process, the board of directors and the new management team were ready to set the direction for ABMH to regain its market leadership position.

Approach and Implementation

Five basic strategies came out of the planning process:

1. Focus on the core business of the hospital—quality patient care.
2. Develop positive medical staff relations and a comprehensive medical staff plan.
3. Control operating expenses.
4. Develop a targeted marketing plan.
5. Develop an effective quality assurance and utilization review program.

Focus on the Core Business of the Hospital—Quality Patient Care

A back-to-basics philosophy was the fundamental strategy driving the new administration. The planning process clearly defined the scope of activities for the hospital in terms of the delivery of health care services. Based on that philosophy, extraneous business lines were divested, sold, or eliminated. The costly Quikcare Card division, designed to facilitate the admissions process, was divested.

Nonperforming assets such as a physician billing service and office buildings were sold. Retail pharmacy businesses were closed. Management contracts for physician practices were terminated. During this phase it was clearly communicated to medical staff, employees, and other relevant audiences that Bergan Mercy was in the business of providing high-quality health care to patients, not in the real estate business, the retail pharmacy business, or the business of practicing medicine. This narrower focus allowed Bergan Mercy to concentrate its resources on the base business, then restore inpatient and outpatient services to a more solid financial footing.

Once some stability was restored to the core hospital business, new ventures and opportunities were analyzed in the context of their contribution to the base business. Those that did not relate directly or contribute to hospital inpatient or outpatient revenues were not undertaken.

Hospital services were grouped into product lines, and a limited number with high growth potential were selected for active development. Four of these areas offered growth opportunities, and these would receive the greatest concentration of management effort and financial resources. They included oncology, orthopedics, obstetrics and gynecology, and cardiology. Communication to medical staff and employees was critical. Employees were able to accept and support the priorities of the hospital, and the net effect of this first strategy was that Bergan Mercy stopped trying to be all things to all people and concentrated on doing a few things very well.

Develop Positive Medical Staff Relations

The diversification and expansion strategies in the mid-1980s had resulted in a deeply divided medical staff. No formal medical staff development plan was in place. The recruitment of physicians was sporadic, and a growing number of the primary care physicians were reaching retirement age. There were gaps in certain specialties. The most serious problem, however, was a sense of distrust among physicians of hospital administration. Physicians perceived inequitable treatment, special deals, and favoritism.

The first step was to set a clear understanding that the hospital was not interested in owning or controlling physician practices. The existing arrangements would be phased out.

The next step was to identify the hospital's vulnerabilities in the medical staff mix and establish guidelines for hospital support in the recruitment or start-up of new physicians. These policies were openly communicated to the staff and were approved by the hospital medical executive committee.

The third step was to prioritize recruitment needs so that the medical staff understood which specialty areas were likely to receive assistance and what form the assistance would take. Administration asked each medical staff department to address the issue of recruitment, and each were given guidelines from the physician staffing plan. Each department was told that the hospital would provide recruitment guarantees not to exceed $30,000 per physician. Some departments chose to initiate recruiting activities, and some did not. This medical staff development plan went a long way toward establishing a foundation of equal and open communication.

Other actions were taken to involve the medical staff in decision making. The hospital board of directors was revamped, and three physicians were added to the eight-member board. Physician representation was implemented at all levels of hospital planning. The medical staff nominating committee selected four physicians for each board position. Then the medical staff voted to select two for each position. The hospital board then reviewed the top two vote getters and selected one of the top two for each position.

The most effective action in turning medical staff relations around, however, was the open communication policy implemented by the entire management team. Management viewed the medical staff as partners, not adversaries. Policy issues, new service issues, or any other matter affecting the medical staff and the hospital were openly communicated. The hospital president individually met with each member of the medical staff to discuss issues and problems. Some physicians reported that it was the first time they ever met face to face with the administrator at Bergan. In two years, the medical staff went from one of the most fragmented to one of the most cohesive in Omaha. Recruitment efforts were very successful, with seven new physicians added to the staff contributing 450 new admissions to the hospital in their first year on staff.

Control Operating Expenses

Integral to the long-term success of the hospital was the strategy of maintaining a position as a high-quality, low-cost provider. To maintain a competitive cost structure, operating expenses were constantly challenged and reduced. Given the shrinking reimbursement climate and a shrinking market, the hospital would need to continually strive for efficiencies in operation.

Actions were taken to achieve economies of scale within the three-hospital system, between ABMH; Mercy Hospital, Council Bluffs, Iowa; and Mercy Hospital, Corning, Iowa. Finance and computer functions were consolidated between the hospitals and duplication in support services like purchasing, central services, and dietary was reduced. Some additional FTE positions were eliminated, although not in patient care areas, bringing the total complement of FTEs to 1,311 in fiscal year 1987, a reduction of 325 from two years before.[7]

Develop a Targeted Marketing Plan

As with most hospitals in a competitive environment, Bergan Mercy looked to the new arena of marketing to solidify its position. Bergan Mercy first used an all-encompassing approach to marketing and advertising, with print and media campaigns aimed at overall image enhancement. Marketing costs were high with few visible results. Since then a more focused approach was developed, aimed at specific audiences. Bergan Mercy's audiences, in order of priority, were identified as (1) physicians, (2) managed care buyers, (3) consumers, and (4) referral agencies or related groups. With the highest priority audience being physicians, a much less costly, more focused marketing approach could be used. Direct, personal contact was selected as the optimum method for reaching this audience, supported by print material such as brochures. Media advertising was eliminated, with the exception of a limited campaign for the hospital's physician referral service. Marketing and advertising expenses went from over $800,000 in 1985 to $200,000 in 1988.

One area where staff was added was in the medical support office, which at Bergan is called the Management Admissions Coordinator (MAC) Department. This office has responsibility for facilitating physician inpatient and outpatient admissions. Its job is to simplify the process for the patient, the physician, and the physician's office staff, while meeting the requirements of the insurance carrier. Three registered nurses were added with sole responsibility for physician marketing and communication. These individuals call on physician offices to communicate new programs and to encourage hospital utilization. The MAC representatives also act as liaisons between the physician and administration in following up on problems or physician concerns. The success of the program stems from the fact that these marketing representatives are nurses who understand the clinical concerns of the physician and the physician's office staff but who also possess superior interpersonal and communication skills. The MAC marketing campaign has been very successful, with an average 20 percent increase in inpatient admissions from those physicians actively called on in fiscal year 1989.

Develop an Effective Quality Assurance and Utilization Program

The quality assurance and utilization review area was strengthened. New software was purchased, and a concentrated effort was made to educate physicians and employees on appropriate utilization. The improved medical staff environment made this a little easier, but it continues to be an area that requires ongoing education and communication. The initial effort was successful. Length of stay for acute inpatients dropped from 6.1 days in 1985 to 5.6 days in fiscal year 1989. With over 80 percent of hospital inpatients under a fixed reimbursement format, it is estimated that the reduction in length of stay equates to an additional $100,000 to the bottom line for every one-tenth reduction.

A specific example of how this reduction was accomplished is in the area of quality assurance and utilization review. The medical staff was able to reduce the length of stay for surgical patients by admitting the patient on the same day surgery is scheduled, instead of the day before. In 1987, on average, the hospital had 90 patient days per month from surgical patients admitted one day before surgery. In 1988, this was reduced to less than 30. The same experience applied to unnecessary days at the end of hospital stays. In this case, the reduction went from an average of 38 unnecessary days per month to less than five. The key factor in implementing the admissions the same day of surgery was the admitting department, which worked closely with physician offices.

External Factors Affecting the Turnaround

Other external factors contributed to Bergan Mercy's turnaround. Bergan Mercy has been very successful in managed care contracting. The trend in the Omaha managed care market is for buyers to contract with a limited number of hospitals, and Bergan Mercy has been successful in negotiating with managed care. This has caused some volume to be diverted to Bergan Mercy from physicians that did not normally use the hospital.

The media was not the hospital's ally during the time of our financial problems. The downsizing that occurred in 1986 received significant, negative press coverage because it was one of the first experienced by Omaha hospitals. While ultimately successful, the hospital was involved in a lengthy, controversial certificate-of-need struggle over open-heart surgery, which also generated negative publicity. The negative publicity did not affect the hospital's ability to accomplish the turnaround, but it did create some fires that diverted management and employees from the task at hand—delivering high-quality services.

It should be noted that the struggle to do open-heart surgery had been going on for almost ten years and was finally approved. In the first year after its approval, more than 200 open-heart procedures were performed and added significantly to the hospital's revenues in 1990.

Hindsight

In retrospect, it was a combination of strategic planning, hard work, and luck that effected the turnaround. The single most important action was the involvement of medical staff in planning and decision making. By making physicians allies of the hospital, the turnaround was able to occur much quicker than anyone thought possible. Physician involvement—in planning meetings, in board meetings, in recruitment, in managed care contracting—is time consuming and often frustrating. It is difficult to obtain consensus from such a fragmented body with often conflicting interests. But the payback in terms of commitment to the hospital is evident.

Remaining Challenges

The turnaround exceeded the expectations of management and the board. Table 7.1 shows the detailed financial performance for each year from 1986 to 1989 for the Omaha Division of Mercy Midlands, which ABMH is a part of. The challenge is to maintain the momentum and to keep the focus on continually improving the quality of services and the efficiency of operations. The obvious changes to realize gains in efficiency have been done (i.e., quality assurance, the consolidation of duplicative departments, etc.). From this point on, it is more difficult to achieve gains. A whole new way of thinking needs to be infused in hospital employees and medical staff. Management and staff have to find ways to do things better, to permanently change the way health care is delivered. If the hospital does

Table 7.1 Revenue and Expense Statement (in thousands)

	1989	1988	1987	1986
Room, board, and nursing care for inpatients	$25,043	$23,167	$23,587	$24,303
Tests, exams, supplies, treatments, and drugs for inpatients	51,810	42,708	37,053	36,334
Nursing care, tests, exams, supplies, treatments, and drugs for outpatients	20,316	16,147	14,207	11,251
Total charges for patient services	$97,169	$82,022	$74,847	$71,888
Less amounts not collected for patient services	22,071	15,878	12,306	10,118
Net amount earned from patient services	$75,098	$66,144	$62,541	$61,770
Other revenue from nonpatient services	2,668	2,488	3,147	2,857
Total revenue	$77,766	$68,632	$65,688	$64,627
Salaries and employee benefits	$36,231	$33,588	$33,198	$36,200
Supplies and purchased services	26,931	22,060	21,617	24,676
Depreciation	4,424	3,909	4,037	4,013
Interest and amortization	2,120	2,137	2,171	2,148
Total operating expenses	$69,706	$61,694	$61,059	$67,037
Net operating income	$ 8,060	$ 6,938	$ 4,629	($ 2,410)
Nonoperating revenues	$ 2,116	$ 1,086	$ 1,158	$ 926
Extraordinary credit (net gain on early extinguishment of debt)				341
Loss on the disposal of discontinued operations and the disposal of a division*			(796)	(253)
Net income	$10,176	$ 8,024	$ 4,991	($ 1,396)

*This income statement reflects income and expenses of the Omaha Division of Mercy Midlands, of which Archbishop Bergan Mercy Hospital is a part.

not continue to innovate and lapses back into past ways of doing things, the ground it has gained will be lost. After a good year, employees and medical staff tend to relax, to stop thinking critically about expense controls, and to let costs creep up again. The challenge is to maintain the enthusiasm and pride the turnaround generated in employees with the innovation, diligence, and attention to costs that fostered the turnaround. Health care continues to be an unforgiving environment for now. The management team believes it has emerged wiser as well as stronger from the turnaround, and it is confident that Bergan Mercy will be not just a survivor but a leader in the provision of health care services to the Omaha community in the years to come.

Notes

1. American Hospital Association, *Economic Trends*, Spring 1989, p. 2.
2. State of Nebraska Department of Health, 1310 Reports, July 1984–June 1986.
3. Ibid., January 1984–June 1988.
4. Ibid.
5. Ibid., July 1988–June 1989.

8

LEADERSHIP TECHNIQUES

Daniel J. Rissing

Editors' Note: The leadership techniques used with most of the various publics of the hospital are described in this chapter. Special attention is paid to correcting physical plant problems, communicating with employees, and the value of a customer orientation. The qualities expected of all managers in a turnaround are clearly outlined and are both valid and invaluable in any kind of turnaround. In addition, the importance of having every employee be able to articulate what needed to be done and of communication with employees is emphasized. This chapter represents a sound, broad-based turnaround of a medium-sized health care institution.

The Market

Zanesville, Ohio, is a community of about 40,000 just one hour east of Columbus, Ohio. The city is a service center for a predominantly rural population of 275,000. Zanesville is an economic hub—county seat, industrial center, and trading point—for a three-county area.

One hundred fifty manufacturing and processing businesses in the area produce a wide variety of products from agricultural machinery to decorative baskets. The area has eight companies with more than 500 employees and seventeen with between 100 and 500 employees.

County unemployment is 9.9 percent, while state and national unemployment are 7.0 percent and 7.1 percent (as of mid-1992). Median household income in the area was about $20,000.

There are two hospitals in Zanesville: Good Samaritan Medical Center, licensed for 400 beds, and Bethesda, licensed for 340 beds. The turnaround occurred at Good Samaritan, which was the older of the two, located near the original center of the city, and landlocked by houses. Bethesda was a new hospital in a medical park in the northern section of the city. Bethesda had a more modern physical plant, plenty of land, and was located in the path of community growth.

The physician community served both hospitals and numbered 61 doctors. The medical staffs were identical. While medical quality was good, many Zanesville area residents would seek specialty care in Columbus. Zanesville was definitely underserved in secondary and tertiary care.

When the change in CEO occurred at Good Samaritan, Bethesda had a market share of 36 percent; Good Samaritan had a market share of 27 percent. Bethesda was financially healthy; Good Samaritan was losing money. There was little question that Bethesda was the leading hospital in the Zanesville area.

Good Samaritan Medical Center had been founded by the Franciscan Sisters Of Christian Charity in 1895. Until the mid-1970s, the sisters had developed a wonderful record of care and service to the Zanesville area. However, when the new CEO arrived, the hospital had been without a leader for almost two years; it had lost market share, had lost money, had developed physical plant problems, and had weak management.

Good Samaritan was definitely a turnaround challenge.

The First Six Months: Analysis on Charrette

It is a tradition in schools of architecture to put students under the pressure of a deadline. As the deadline for presentation draws near, the students, working with chalk on moveable blackboards known as charrettes, are often making their final lines and calculations as the charrettes are being pushed down the hall to a jury of faculty members. It is drawing on charrette, analysis on the run.

Good Samaritan's dismal financial picture necessitated an analysis of the market and the hospital on the run—on charrette. It was apparent there would not be the luxury of a one- to two-year planning hiatus or a gradual and comfortable learning curve. For all the risks associated with analysis on the run, there was an immediate need for action and improvement.

In the early moments of this assignment, at least eight major areas of concern were identified, which became the focus of the turnaround:

1. No strategic plan in existence, no direction
2. Many interpersonal problems

3. Financial pressure—the hospital was losing money and financial controls were weak

4. Serious physical plant problems

5. Unmet health needs in the market

6. Weak leadership and management

7. A culture without an orientation to the customer

8. Declining market share, a lack of community support

The eight issues became the basis for long-term goals that guided everything the administration did to return Good Samaritan to good health. The following discussion describes the tactics that resulted in success.

Building Interpersonal Bridges: Communication, Communication, and More Communication

In the CEO's interview for the Good Samaritan assignment, it became clear that doctors, board members, managers, and employees were not in touch with one another. Everyone had bits and pieces of information, and no one seemed to have the entire picture. There was little trust. There was a substantial gap between the hospital and the community. The CEO needed to build bridges quickly or the organization would not repair, heal, and excel.

The CEO's first day on the job began what would prove to be a nonstop series of meetings: one-on-one sessions with board members, the top 25 medical staff admitters, and every middle manager and top manager. The conversations were mostly one way: they did most of the talking.

Following these meetings, another series of meetings with all employees was held, and the CEO began making rounds on each shift to personally meet each of the 1,200 employees.

At this stage, the CEO had to spend long hours inside the hospital, to hand out in the doctors lounge, and to make regular rounds. A typical day began at five or six in the morning and ended late at night. It was necessary to work at this contact and visibility for about five months, setting an example for the other leaders and managers.

The administration also initiated a series of meetings with community leaders in the early days. The meetings took the form of focus groups and provided marketing research.

What must a leader do in the first six months of a new challenge? A leader must establish a style and a set of values that begin to form a desired culture. The message, by example, was clear to all: open, solid, and frequent communication was expected from every person to every other person. Personal concern for the individual and strong cooperation person-to-person and department-to-department was to become the rule. The fastest way to establish the values was to demonstrate them. At Good Samaritan the CEO maintained this style of visibility and frequent contact throughout his tenure. His personal goal was to always be in touch with the board, employees, physicians, patients, managers, and the community.

Medical staff. The doctors were concerned about survival. There were no funds for education or the improvement of employee clinical skills, much less for technological advances. They reported that the building and equipment had been ignored for some time.

Top and middle management. The managers had been without a leader for a long time. They were unsure of the future. Honesty and trust were in question. Many were concerned about and even fearful of the marginal performance of some of their colleagues in recent years.

Employees. Employees had grave concerns about basic questions like, Will we get a paycheck next week? Will we survive? Is the hospital going to be around next year? They did not think that management cared about them or listened to them. These were typical statements in the early employee meetings.

The community. Feedback from community leaders revealed that Bethesda owned the high-technology position in the market. Good Samaritan was considered the high-touch hospital that had slipped a bit in recent years. The sentiment seemed to be that Good Samaritan would be warm and friendly, but anyone who was really sick would not want to go there.

The sisters had earned high regard in the community among Protestants and Catholics for their decades of sacrifice and human service. Community leaders viewed the hospital as a major factor in the economy. As the hospital began community meetings outside of Zanesville, it learned that it had more support outside the city than in it.

Leadership Technique: Weekly Community Forums

Among the many successful bridge-building techniques implemented was the weekly community forum. The hospital began by inviting the political representatives to the hospital for lunch and, with their help, began to build a list of names of people to include in future meetings. A personal invitation signed by the president would go out with a simple agenda: come, meet with us, and tell us how we are doing and what we could do better. Following the meeting the hospital took care to send a personal thank-you note to each person—always timely, always personal.

The program was well received and so helpful that the hospital extended it to the countryside. It assigned a manager or vice president to each community in the area. It was the manager's job to coordinate programs for area leaders in the region.

Gradually, taking programs to the rural communities enabled the hospital to establish close relationships with area residents. It was able to bring the best of these residents onto the newly formed associate board, where the hospital kept them apprised of ideas and developments. This approach is strongly recommended, for it has multiple benefits, including

- accurate and timely health delivery feedback from all sectors,
- community exposure for middle management,
- a mechanism to reaffirm the hospital's mission and strategic direction, and
- dialogue with and development of friends of the hospital.

The Reason Many Organizations Fail to Implement Their Plans: They Do Not Have Any Plans

What a surprise it was to find that Good Samaritan did not have a formal strategic plan. There was no direction. It soon became apparent that the organization did not know how to plan, and there was no one on board who could lead this important work. Without a plan or planning sensitivity, serious errors can occur. And they did.

An attached physicians office building had been constructed without a certificate of need. A radiology special procedures room had been constructed without a certificate of need. To add insult to injury, the equipment for the room had been received and paid for a year earlier but had not been installed.

In the bridge-building process with the board members, the administration quickly achieved consensus that a plan was needed and that it would attempt a fast-track planning process.

Leadership Technique: The Selection of a Planning Consultant

To expedite things, the CEO took a small risk and did not search for proposals for planning assistance. He hired a known entity, someone he had worked with successfully in the past, and began sessions with the board, medical staff leadership, and management on the planning process. In effect, the CEO tested the acceptance of the consultant, looked for good chemistry in these early educational meetings, and found it. The administration then proceeded to develop a plan. Had the CEO not found good chemistry or acceptance, he would have backed off and gone the traditional route of a request for proposals and qualifying interviews. This technique saved a great deal of time.

Working with a new board-level planning committee, the administration began working on the plan. There was a clear theme: the plan would drive the budget. Any planning that had been done in the past at Good Samaritan was driven by the need for a budget.

The process really gave us three plans: a program plan, a facilities plan, and a site plan. The latter was important since the hospital was nearly landlocked.

The other theme of the planning process was involvement. The administration involved board members, doctors, management, employees, the mother house, and community residents. Pushing as hard as it could, it developed a plan. But in many ways, the plan was a by-product of the process. The real valued outcome was a commitment on a direction, a real measure of consensus, and stronger relationships between the players.

The plan gave the hospital the following direction:

- Develop centers of excellence. Responsibility for select service lines, particularly those that had high profit margins or high volumes, was assigned to various members of the administrative staff. Each center then developed its own objectives, and some even had their own logos.
- Continue planning with the medical staff. The medical staff actually developed their own plan for the improvement of the hospital. That plan was submitted to the hospital's planning committee, and positions were integrated into the hospital's long-range plan.
- Develop a construction program to improve the building. The hospital had no master facility plan but began developing a 30-year master plan. A program to upgrade all major inpatient and out-

patient care areas (70 percent of the building) was immediately begun. These improvements had a positive effect on employees as well as patients.

- Put $280,000 profit on the books as soon as possible. This goal was reached by improving efficiencies. There were no layoffs or downsizing during this stage.
- Increase market share by 5 percent. This goal was accomplished through focused marketing programs.
- Recruit physicians. A formal physician staffing plan was developed and endorsed. Most of the recruitment was done in conjunction with existing physicians. The result was a doubling of the size of the medical staff in three years.
- Improve customer satisfaction. The hospital established ongoing customer satisfaction surveys in outpatient and inpatient areas. In addition, major customer satisfaction surveys were done twice annually.

Perhaps the most important thing the administration did was to make a conscious effort to create a high level of understanding for what it was going to do. The goal was for every employee to be able to articulate what the hospital was going to do. To achieve this goal necessitated another series of employee meetings. These really became annual state of the organization meetings. Obviously, the information about the hospital's plans would get to the competition, but that did not matter. To move ahead successfully, everyone on the team must understand the plan and support it. The administration worked hard on this point, and if any employee was stopped in the hall and asked what the hospital was committed to do, he or she could answer point by point.

Participation in the employee meetings was slow at first. They were new to the process and not very trusting. After the second phase of meetings, participation picked up. One employee said, "We never had the chance before to talk with the CEO, to be included as part of a team, or to make suggestions. It never happened in the past."

The Financial Picture:
The Hospital Could Not Buy a Bucket of Paint

The financial picture at Good Samaritan was bleak. The hospital had lost money or broken even for years. The first year after the new CEO came, it lost $600,000. Things were so bad, it could not buy a bucket of paint.

When the hospital developed construction plans, it needed $100,000 for owner's equity in the project. It had to borrow all of it.

The attack on the financial problems consisted of five basic tactics:

1. Make everyone more efficient and careful with scarce resources. People had to become more accountable.
2. Obtain rate increases as appropriate. Good Samaritan was one of the low-cost hospitals in the state, but it was not developing enough revenue.
3. Improve the physical plant to enable the hospital to attract new and additional business.
4. Employ the concept of funded depreciation and reinvest the funds.
5. Ask the medical staff for more referrals.

Leadership Technique: Ask for the Business

When the change in CEO at Good Samaritan occurred, occupancy was at 42 percent. It was a going broke. The doctors were mostly going to the competitor, Bethesda. They had little confidence in Good Samaritan and no real allegiance. The physician customer was mostly supporting the competition.

The medical staff was addressed at every opportunity, formally and informally, and asked for their business. We appealed to them as candidly as possible: If you value a two-hospital system in Zanesville, then you must begin to support Good Samaritan. We want your referrals and we wantmore balance in your referrals. If you do not give us the business, we will fail.

In return, they received a promise to improve the quality of care using increased and improved education and training. They responded well to the appeal, and things began to improve.

The five tactics paid off. Good Samaritan began to make a profit and continued to be profitable every year after that.

Physical Plant Improvements: A Four-Year Chess Game

The Good Samaritan physical plant had been neglected. As soon as possible, the administration began what turned out to be a four-year chess game in which almost every department moved once. The hospital had insufficient private rooms and was still operating three- and four-bed wards.

The buildings that made up the physical plant were well maintained in many cases, but they were old, designed and built for a different era.

The hospital had boilers from the 1930s and 1940s, and the laundry was so old it could have been depreciated four or five times. Surgery facilities were antiquated, air handling was poor, the hospital could not maintain temperature or humidity in the operating rooms, special care was underbedded and too far from surgery, the radiology and laboratory departments were out of date, and facilities for patients, families, doctors, and employees were unpleasant.

Thirty different departments were totally changed or improved in a major way within four years. For example, the administration worked with the users—both physicians and operating room technicians—and with inpatients and outpatients to redesign the operating room suites. The result was a tripling in the size of the operating room area and significant improvements in the efficiencies of the entire department.

Leadership Technique: Motivating Your People While Putting Them through Constant Change

While the construction projects were designed to improve conditions for the employees as well as the customers, it became clear that motivation was necessary to maintain morale in the face of tremendous change. It is undeniable that change, even if it is in one's best interests, is a negative idea for many and upsetting for most. Our people would have to live with constant change for at least four years.

To combat resistance to change and the unsettling effect constant change can have on a service organization, conscious plans were developed to ease the stress. Employee communication was given a high priority. Involvement was a major theme during the physical plant renovations. Departments and doctors were heavily involved in planning. Once designs were complete, the hospital would mock up a department with masking tape on the floor of an old gym to show spacial relationships. Sometimes it actually constructed cardboard walls to allow people to walk through the spaces they would work in. When a new department finally emerged from the dust and din, the hospital showcased the improvements and changes and celebrated another victory. After four years, the hospital had a physical plant that was up to date, functioned well, and was competitive.

The bond issue was made through a public offering after a detailed financial feasibility study was completed. Total long-term debt at the facility amounted to $35,000,000 after the bond issue.

Construction costs ultimately totaled $15,000,000 and were funded by a bond issue.

Meeting Unmet Health Care Needs:
Doctors and Information

The unmet health needs of the Zanesville area fell into two categories: a lack of physicians and a lack of community information about health issues and solutions.

Primary care in the area was not well staffed. At one time there were three dozen primary care doctors in the region, but the numbers had dropped to six. Doctors were not being replaced, and our regional feeder mechanism was in trouble. Specialties were also deficient. Many people were leaving the area for secondary and tertiary care. Columbus is a major medical center and is an easy drive from Zanesville.

The hospital began recruiting. It urged its doctors to recruit, it recruited, and it helped the doctors in any way possible. The net result was a tripling of the medical staff in ten years, and in the process, the average age of the staff was lowered from 58 to 39. Among the specialties recruited: hematology and oncology, pulmonary, vascular surgery, obstetrics, neurosurgery, general surgery, ear, nose, and throat (ENT), plastic surgery, cardiology, pediatrics, general internal medicine, and primary care doctors for rural communities.

An outside firm was not used for recruitment. Moreover, giveaways were not part of the program. Payment for office start-ups and assistance in establishing practices in surrounding communities were used with great success.

At Good Samaritan, major improvements were made in the following services: obstetrics and gynecology, cancer, emergency, pediatrics, and radiation therapy. The surgery department in general, intensive care, and outpatient services received major focus.

To improve community understanding and to promote the acceptance of new and existing services, the hospital began pumping information into the community. It developed aggressive publicity to support the improvements and developed screening and health education programs to teach people about health problems and acquaint them with the solutions.

Leadership Technique: Team Building and Values

When people live with problems long enough, they begin to accept them. The problems and deficiencies become part of the landscape. To an outsider, the problems were mostly clear and easy to spot. In the early days for the new CEO, people had to be convinced that things were not right and could certainly be greatly improved.

The board had fallen into an operating trap: they were involved in day-to-day operating decisions. In many ways, management and leadership found it easier to defer to the board. Board members, feeling their stewardship responsibilities, jumped in and tried to improve things. The board was managing, and the managers were asleep. This process had been in effect for more than two years.

Once the roles were straightened out and the board was back to a policy-setting mode, the CEO had to tackle the management team.

Certain qualities were clearly expected in all managers:

- They must be committed to the turnaround.
- They must embrace change.
- There must be no Green Berets, only team players.
- They must lead as well as manage.
- They must have good work ethics and lead by example.
- They must work well with doctors.
- They must be consistent and steady.
- They must be positive.

What followed then was a sorting process. Of the 34 people in upper management, the administration replaced 22. Three of the managers assumed new positions.

To develop skills, the hospital introduced a training program that began with monthly management meetings from two to three hours in length. About one-third of the meeting was given to education. The hospital also began an annual retreat in which management left the hospital and worked together for a day or two in an attempt to strengthen its team building.

To help form the desired management culture, the administration constantly solicited input, encouraged them to participate, and expected them to communicate openly and regularly.

The fact that the administration was able to restore the health of Good Samaritan Medical Center is a direct result of the efforts of the management group that emerged. They were given the opportunity, and they delivered. Let there be no mistake: the turnaround of Good Samaritan was only possible because of the tremendous combined effort of employees, physicians, managers, board members, and the sisters. A turnaround is not possible unless such cooperation exists.

The Concept of the Customer and
the Value of Promotion

The concept of the customer emerged in the health care world in the 1970s. Like most hospitals, Good Samaritan had a patient orientation and a concern with good diagnosis and treatment. The culture was clinically oriented. It became clear that a customer orientation had to develop if it was to be competitive.

The hospital introduced the concept of the customer through a customer service training program. The program was a beginning and not a panacea. The program also had to belong to the hospital. It developed a cadre of employee trainers and carefully asked its people to consider the concept of the customer. It was stressed that customers were people who made purchasing decisions, who made choices. They could choose Good Samaritan or they could choose our competitor. The administration let the employees define who the customer were, and they did it well. The hospital emphasized customer satisfaction as an important key to its survival and prosperity.

To reinforce the concept, the hospital conducted numerous ongoing customer surveys. It surveyed the patients, the medical staff, and the residents of the market. The hospital demonstrated that it would try to measure its performance and that every employee was responsible for the customers' perception of satisfaction.

Good Samaritan had been reluctant to promote its services or even its presence. It realized that in competitive times, advertising is essential.

After careful consideration, the hospital selected a theme that was based on its past and who it was. The theme was "Your Care Is Our Tradition." In many ways, it suggested the tremendous contribution the sisters had made to the community. The hospital developed an advertising campaign to introduce the theme and then developed product-specific advertisements to follow the introduction. The hospital elected to use print, television, billboards, and radio. As the process unfolded, the hospital realized that its identity program was dated. It developed and prepared a new logo and signature to fit the new mood of the organization.

In keeping with the hospital's style and culture, the administration did nothing with the program until the employees and managers agreed it was fitting and would support it. The hospital held a series of employee meetings and shared what had been developed. The staff was told that if they could not support the messages, they would not work. The hospital received a great deal of support from its family, and some even seemed relieved that the hospital was going to be aggressive. It was felt that the promotion was effective from the standpoint of developing business and positioning Good Samaritan as an upbeat, technically progressive, and caring place.

In Retrospect: What Would We Improve?

Looking back, two things might have been improved:

1. The hospital should have done everything sooner.
2. It should have worked harder to build a Good Samaritan medical staff.

The medical staff was composed of some wonderful doctors, but they tried to straddle the competition issue. The two hospitals in town had essentially the same medical staff. Most of the doctors tried to be balanced in their approach to admissions. If Bethesda pushed them, they moved in its direction. If Good Samaritan pushed them, they moved in its direction. In retrospect, Good Samaritan should have worked harder to build its own medical staff. It is difficult, at best, to run a business in a competitive market without loyal and committed customers.

The Good Samaritan Medical Center turnaround produced some solid results:

- There was a sense of team and family inside the hospital. Spirit returned.
- The community now views Good Samaritan as the emerging leader in health care.
- Market share increased from 27 percent to 37 percent.
- Good Samaritan made a profit in the second year of the turnaround and every year after that for 10 years.
- Continual surveys show a high level of customer satisfaction with the hospital's people and services.
- Good Samaritan is a leader in community health education in the Zanesville area. It was the first hospital in Ohio to install TelMed. It created a brown bag lunch forum in which local residents could attend a program at noon on an endless variety of health care subjects. Most were held at the hospital. Poison control kits were

distributed through the emergency room and a Family Walk and Fun Run was developed to promote good health and raise funds for the hospital.

- The hospital developed a hospice and took wellness and industrial medicine programs to area businesses.
- An active foundation was established to create giving opportunities for area residents.
- A Good Samaritan center of excellence, in physical medicine and rehabilitation, formed the basis for a for-profit venture that began as consulting and certificate-of-need assistance and then led to actual program development for other hospitals, culminating in the actual design and construction of free-standing rehabilitation hospitals in Kentucky and West Virginia.
- The year before the turnaround was initiated, the hospital lost approximately $600,000. The next year it had a surplus from operations of $800,000. The second and third years of the turnaround resulted in surpluses of $1.2 million and $1 million respectively.

Fond Memories of Fine People

Looking back, the lesson is clear: the people are the product. Without the dedication and support of hundreds of fellow employees, little would have been accomplished; the Good Samaritan turnaround would not have happened.

The most important achievement in Zanesville is the knowledge that teams of health care workers at Good Samaritan Medical Center are now taking good care of patients. The spirit and substance of patient care is alive and well at Good Samaritan.

9

THE LONG VIEW

John E. Friedlander and Charles H. Kachmarik, Jr.

Editors' Note: This chapter focuses on both the expense portion and revenue portion of the turnaround equation. It focuses on the decline of the organization before the process that was instituted to turn the hospital around. The chapter also describes the corporate restructuring of the hospital to give it additional flexibility and the diversification into a small health care system from a single, stand-alone institution. The financial results of the efforts are described over about eight years. The turnaround chronicled in this chapter is the longest described in this book.

In current health care jargon, a *hospital turnaround* is thought of as a situation in which a significant set of hospital problems, perhaps chronic, are addressed through a process involving a variety of groups and disciplines. One can generally attribute a well-defined time period to the turnaround, perhaps as much as four to six years, after which definitive results can be seen, outcomes measured, and a reshaped institutional direction established.

It is certain that every hospital turnaround is different. The uniqueness of the Buffalo General Hospital (BGH) turnaround lies in the broad vision, of what BGH could become, the precedents set to achieve that vision, and the ability of a hospital board and management to sustain success over a 15-year period.

The events one can now, in retrospect, call the BGH turnaround can be divided into three stages, each serving as a building block for the next, without which the subsequent stage could not have occurred.

The Vision: 1975 to 1982

In 1975, BGH was a 750-bed private, acute care teaching hospital that maintained, as it does today, a primary teaching affiliation with the State University of New York at Buffalo (SUNY@B) School of Medicine.

A young physician-administrator named William V. Kinnard, Jr., M.D., had just assumed the position of the hospital's president and CEO. He came to BGH with an expansive vision, a vision shared by his predecessor and the board of trustees: For the hospital to continue its success in clinical care, serve as the region's major tertiary care hospital, and carry out its academic and research activities, it must be completely expanded and restored.

A deteriorating hospital structure had begun to seriously undermine the ability of physicians to adequately care for patients in outdated facilities using antiquated equipment. Patients, in increasing numbers, expressed great reluctance to be hospitalized in such facilities; only the outstanding care physicians and nurses delivered continued to draw patients.

In addition to patient and physician perceptions of the facilities, hospital management was increasingly frustrated with its inability to operate cost-efficiently and effectively. On every front, by 1975 Buffalo General was at an increasingly clear competitive disadvantage. Thus, Kinnard began to articulate his vision, which can be captured in one of his most succinct statements: No longer could Buck Rogers medicine be practiced in Civil War facilities. His vision of a new Buffalo General was an expansive one, one swiftly adopted by the internal hospital family.

While the vision of a new Buffalo General was affirmed time and again, the linchpin of the turnaround, new hospital facilities, was not immediately achievable. Other constituencies had to be involved in a project of this magnitude. The planning process, or as Kinnard is fond of saying, "the reconciliation of perspectives," had to be moved forward. Between 1976 and 1979, community leaders, legislative and government officials, health planners, and many others nominated various options to achieve the BGH vision. The hospital tried but failed to avoid the duplication of construction efforts with the County Hospital Authority as it contemplated major hospital construction. Programs of significant downsizing, along with various hospital merger strategies, were suggested as alternatives to Buffalo General's massive rebuilding effort; however, each seemed to offer substantially more risk than benefit to the community.

By 1979, one strategy did survive that served to sustain the vision. This strategy offered the possibility of merging the financially unstable

362-bed Deaconess Hospital with the 750-bed Buffalo General. Since Deaconess was within one mile of BGH, it was felt that a merged entity would preserve sufficient acute care beds to serve the community's needs and reduce program and service duplication while enhancing programs and services necessary to address the area's unique needs. Deaconess Hospital would ultimately be converted to a health care center that would house skilled nursing home beds on the top floors and primary ambulatory care services on the lower ones.

The vision now had substantial form, substance, and acceptance, both with the hospital family and important community constituencies (including the Western New York Health Services Administration (HSA); since the HSA would play a significant role in the approval process, it was consistently kept abreast of the hospital's plans). Without this level of acceptance, the turnaround process would not have moved forward.

The hospital's vision required approval by the Western New York HSA and both the state and federal government. A major effort was necessary to package the vision to be easily understood and interpreted by planning and regulatory bodies to obtain approval for construction and financing.

The hospital's team of experts included, among others, Coopers & Lybrand and Merrill Lynch. Both firms have played an integral part in the 15-year turnaround but no more important a role than during the first stage.

Beginning in late 1979, Coopers & Lybrand staff provided the hospital's strategic financial and planning direction throughout the state and federal regulatory review process. The strategy was apparent: without expansion and renovation, the hospital was sure to see decreasing physician use, occupancy decline, growing expense for operating an outdated plant, and ultimately an inability to carry out the institution's mission. Coopers & Lybrand's demand and financial forecasts projected growth and opportunity after 1985 when the new facility was completed, yet it would take major financing, estimated to be in excess of $200 million, to achieve this goal. Financing of this magnitude required the expertise of a firm dealing in the field of hospital debt financing. Merrill Lynch was selected for this task. The hospital's expert team was complete and ready to face the challenge of final approval.

With the HSA's involvement in and understanding of the hospital's vision, the planning agency easily adopted the concepts embodied in the institution's mission and helped to convey them to the broader constituency throughout the Western New York eight-county planning region.

The New York State Health Department had been involved in the consideration of various community-hospital strategies since 1976. Early in the vision's formulation, the hospital and health department officials worked closely to achieve a responsible plan for rebuilding Buffalo General while ensuring the proper balance of beds, programs, and services for the community. The health department had the vision in place when Deaconess Hospital was guided into the merger with Buffalo General in 1979.

The federal government became critically important as the vision gained wider acceptance. The Departments of Health and Human Services (HHS) and Housing and Urban Development (HUD) have made available to hospitals and nursing homes a federally guaranteed mortgage program to obtain financing when, on the basis of a facility's financial strength, assurances of debt repayment were limited. Historically, most hospitals in New York State have had that problem due to stringent reimbursement regulations. After two years of plan review, the federal government agreed to guarantee a $210 million capital financing under the FHA-242 Program. It was the largest hospital financing ever guaranteed by Washington to that point and has only recently been eclipsed by two other New York City hospital projects.

By 1982, the vision had become reality. The renovation and expansion of Buffalo General was about to commence. The first stage of the hospital's turnaround as we know it today was complete, but only then did the hospital begin to experience problems that would shake the foundation of the vision and that would characterize the second major stage of the turnaround.

Implementation: 1982 to 1984

One of the largest hospital bond issues ever sold in the United States was closed in October 1982, a year that was marked by major change in Western New York.

In the midst of making the hospital's vision a reality and establishing a bright and progressive future, Buffalo General found itself in a region that was under economic and demographic siege. This siege mentality was exacerbated by the legacy of Buffalo's famous Blizzard of '77.

Since 1977, Buffalo had become the butt of every conceivable story and joke about the weather; it had become the snow capital of the western world. The community collectively suffered a near depression and a temporary loss of pride in the strongly held beliefs about the high quality of life in the region. The community psyche had been damaged, and a recovery was not in the foreseeable future. The smokestack industries that contributed to a thriving economy were closing. Major steel plants, such as Bethlehem Steel, employing over 7,000 workers, rapidly closed in 1982. The ancillary businesses designed to supply big steel and other heavy industry were similarly affected. Inflation, increased international competition, and a lack of modern plants and equipment led to the growing demise of the region's economy. The industrial sector, which employed a large portion of the area's population, had simply disappeared.

Along with the loss of industry went the jobs. High unemployment gave rise to additional problems, some of which, to this day, have dramatically and permanently affected Buffalo General. The most significant of these problems included the emigration of a young work force, which increased significantly in the early 1980s. Not only were young working families leaving, but as a result the significant number of elderly remaining in Western New York became more apparent.

In addition to a rapidly emerging elderly population, the region's demographic changes suggested the need for a more well-balanced service-industrial economy, which could not be put in place quickly.

As a major part of the service sector, Buffalo General was back in the community spotlight. The economic changes in Buffalo suggested to many members of the hospital's work force that they could no longer rely simply on the good faith of their employer. Job protection and job security were essential. Additionally, the high inflation years of the Carter and early Reagan administrations, along with a prevailing negative community attitude, had all created the right conditions for a nursing unionization effort. The suggestion that new facilities would bring about operating efficiencies or perhaps a loss of jobs also proved to be a strong signal for proponents of unionization to begin aggressive organizing efforts.

By the end of 1982 and into early 1983, nurse unionization efforts had achieved a high degree of success. Two other unions were already representing small sectors of the hospital's 3,200 employees. Their presence along with the external factors previously discussed enabled a rapid organizing effort to quickly achieve a recognition and representation vote leading to contract negotiations by early summer of 1983.

Construction was underway. The debris and overall disarray that normally accompanies major construction programs was present. Working conditions in the still-occupied buildings continued to deteriorate as the vision of a new Buffalo General was kept alive. Four other key issues that complicated the hospital's operating situation were also emerging.

The 1979 merger plan required the consolidation of Deaconess Hospital into Buffalo General. Concurrent with this undertaking, the planning of a new hospital contemplated the five-year phaseout of Deaconess as an acute care facility. Operating under that assumption, key members of the Deaconess medical staff, beginning in 1980, chose to move their practices elsewhere. A number of orthopedists, obstetricians, internists, and family medicine physicians decided that Buffalo General would be unable to adequately support the increasing financial demands at both sites, plan and construct a new facility, and fully accommodate their needs to be incorporated into a different practice setting from the type they had been practicing. Instead, they chose other community hospitals for their patients. Deaconess was struggling financially at the time of the merger, and the physician relocations further complicated this problem.

In 1978, Deaconess had a loss from operations of $2.9 million. The Deaconess plant required a significant upgrade along with the replacement of major equipment for patient care. In commencing Buffalo General's merger plan, the Deaconess plant would not be immediately renovated. The Deaconess acute care operation continued to contribute to the overall BGH corporate financial instability until 1985 when all acute care services were completely moved to Buffalo General. The State of New York initially provided reimbursement relief to address cash flow problems of the newly merged corporation. This relief positioned Buffalo General to report a 1979 bottom-line gain of $1.3 million on total revenues of $78.8 million. But the effect of this assistance was short-lived as Deaconess physicians began admitting elsewhere and the cost of maintaining two acute care sites dramatically increased. By 1981, the merged Buffalo General/Deaconess Corporation had again begun showing bottom-line losses. The added reimbursement assistance provided by the state had run its course.

Why Deaconess remained open was obviously questioned. The answer was clear. Part of the political support necessary to achieve new hospital construction was achieved through an accommodation between the hospital, the community, and state legislative representatives to keep Deaconess open and accessible as an acute care facility until the new Buffalo General construction was complete. This political accommodation was an element essential to obtaining the support necessary to gain state construction approval. In retrospect, no one had anticipated that the rapid and dramatic changes that occurred at Deaconess would leave it as a poorly occupied, overstaffed, and financially burdensome acute care operation.

Two other events were also on the horizon; both involved nursing but differed in their level of impact on Buffalo General. The first was the role of the Buffalo General Hospital School of Nursing, a diploma program which held the distinction of being the second oldest nursing school in the United States. For many years, it had proudly served as an educational resource for the community and the hospital. This distinction perhaps was its downfall. By 1983 the average class size had substantially declined. The school competed with a number of other diploma and bachelor-degree-granting schools in Western New York. In recent years the number of nursing school programs had increased so that the classes at the BGH program were only 50 percent full, while tuition was kept low for competitive reasons. In addition, critical to the assessment of the school's future was the fact that less than 50 percent of the nurses trained and graduated were retained at Buffalo General for employment; over 50 percent of the hospital's registered nurses were trained elsewhere. The cost of maintaining a high quality faculty and program on limited tuition required that the hospital bear any deficit between tuition and other revenue support and the cost of operating the school. In 1983, the deficit was $500,000, and by 1984 it had reached $750,000. The hospital board and management were compelled to act on this major issue to ensure the hospital's survival.

The other key nursing issue was unionization. By the summer of 1983, labor union recognition had not progressed. Sentiment ran quite high, both at the board and senior management levels, that unionization would have significant repercussions for the future of Buffalo General and other voluntary not-for-profit hospitals in Western New York. It was felt that a firm position on union recognition and negotiation must be taken even if a strike occurred. A nursing strike did occur and did not end for 79 days. It is not necessary to discuss the many heroic and perhaps less than heroic actions that took place. Suffice it to say that the strike proved to be an event that is still all too familiar to many after seven years (particularly since the hospital has, since 1983, recognized the registered nurses as a full-fledged bargaining unit).

Unionization came at a time when Buffalo General was most vulnerable. The hospital's physical plant was being replaced, and hospital operations were highly compromised. While hospital management attempted to operate through the difficulties of construction, the team was simultaneously managing the Deaconess merger. With over 900 nurses on strike for nearly three months, the hospital's vision was fundamentally threatened.

Buffalo General began to hemorrhage financially in 1983 as the cumulative result of these events. An operating loss in excess of $5 million was reported. This situation was virtually unchanged in 1984 with another devastating operating loss of $4.8 million. Nonoperating gains did little to offset the problem, with the hospital reporting bottom-line losses of $4.2 million and $3.1 million respectively.

The nursing strike had soundly but temporarily driven physicians and their patients away from Buffalo General, much the same as at the outset of the Deaconess merger. Ever increasing losses were being experienced through maintaining acute care services at Deaconess Hospital, and other costs such as the mounting deficit in the School of Nursing added to the complexity of the situation. The evolving Buffalo General turnaround now had a more immediate agenda. Operational and financial health had to be preserved while the vision for the future was aggressively pursued.

In 1983, events external to the hospital were no more beneficial. In just nine short months the president, with Congress strongly behind him, passed landmark health care financing legislation. The PPS and DRG system began, and although it did not reach New York State until 1986 when the Medicare waiver expired, the legislation sent a clear message to hospitals and physicians alike that government was going to become an active player in the payment of health care (Medicare and Medicaid) benefits.

The Buffalo General turnaround had been based on the notion that hospital facilities could and should meet the ever increasing demand for inpatient care in a teaching and high technology setting. This was the general philosophy that characterized hospital construction in the late 1970s and early 1980s. Yet, in this rapidly changing regulatory environment and in the course of a major construction effort, significant planning and other assumptions had to be examined, reconsidered, and altered. In 1983, the DRG philosophy shifted the health care system away from per diem payment, where more days of care resulted in more revenue, to one that paid a flat rate for a standardized incident of care with little regard for how many days were required to achieve patient discharge. Buffalo General, like most other hospitals in the United States, had experienced dramatic increases in patient days, reaching a high point in 1980 when the hospital recorded over 337,000 days. The primary justification and premise of financial feasibility for capital construction projects, including this one, was that large numbers of beds were needed to accommodate more patients who each seemed to stay, by today's standards, for excessive periods of time.

By 1984, Buffalo General had experienced a reduction of 81,400 days to 255,600 days of care, maintaining an average length of stay of just over 10 days. At the same time, outpatient and specialized ambulatory care services began to dramatically increase.

A new dimension of leadership was necessary to keep the vision close at hand. New strategies and planning initiatives had to be developed to keep the hospital's direction on track and address these systemic changes. At the same time a significant operational effort was required to move the hospital back to operational and financial stability.

The board of trustees and Kinnard stepped up to this challenge by recognizing that Kinnard could not single-handedly carry the direct leadership responsibility for both efforts. He had to delegate many of the operational turnaround activities to a second in command while he guided the overall direction of the initiative started in 1975.

At the end of 1984, Kinnard appointed the hospital's first executive vice-president and COO (John Friedlander, the hospital's current president and CEO), to assume this major role in the turnaround. The third stage of the evolving turnaround was underway. The vision was within reach, but major obstacles still had to be overcome.

The Turnaround Is Completed:
1984 to the Present Day

While it is likely that no hospital turnaround is ever complete because of the many environmental changes that must be addressed, the last five years at Buffalo General can be viewed as both a conclusion to the vision and a foundation for future visions.

By the latter half of 1984, the cumulative effect of the many hospital events described above was being felt. Between 1982 and 1984, the hospital had a combined bottom-line loss of $11.6 million. The asset base had been substantially reduced by two factors: (1) funds were restricted for use as project equity, and (2) additional cash was required annually during this period to keep the hospital operating. The nurses' strike had paralyzed the institution in 1983, and it was not until early 1984 that the census and full operation began to show signs of recovery. However, it was a very different hospital in 1984. Over 300 FTEs had been eliminated. The occupancy rate, still a crucial measure of success while on a per diem system, had dropped from nearly 89 percent in 1982 to 65 percent in both 1983 and 1984. To sustain daily operations, including meeting payroll, purchasing supplies, and keeping the utilities working, a $5 million unsecured line of credit was obtained—$1 million each from five local banks. The basis for the extension of this credit was that Buffalo General was part of the cultural fabric of the community. A 130-year history was at stake along with a multimillion-dollar replacement of the institution. The

banks could also not ignore that the hospital was the fifth largest employer in Buffalo and that the economy at the time could not tolerate any
more significant financial instability from any sector, including health
care.

The loyalty of the active physicians was strained but not broken.
Many of the physicians had experienced significant interruptions in their
daily practice activities during the nurses' strike. They had expressed
reluctance and concern about the full use of the hospital following the strike
based on fears that their practices might be similarly affected in the future.
They also were unable to understand the hospital's position on unionization. The management team's and the board's credibility was thus at stake
in the physicians' eyes.

An aggressive plan was required by the end of 1984 to operationally
manage the hospital to full recovery. Immediately, strategic, and tactical
directions were developed, which included the following:

- The performance of a broadly based opinion survey to determine
  what three important constituencies—the general public, the
  employees, and the medical staff—thought of the hospital. (There
  were major benefits to doing a self-study at this critical juncture.
  One, it benchmarked where the hospital was with each of the
  constituencies and, as changes were implemented, progress could
  better be judged. The second benefit was that responses to particular
  constituencies could be more sharply focused. Third, it gave each
  group the opportunity to be heard and to feel they had input as this
  phase of the turnaround progressed.)
- Repayment of the $5 million line of credit, restoring a positive cash
  position for the hospital
- The restoration of full involvement by the active medical staff at
  Buffalo General to maintain and ultimately increase hospital
  admissions and ambulatory services utilization
- The expeditious elimination of the major financial drains on the
  hospital, particularly the Deaconess acute care operation and the
  school of nursing
- The establishment of a break-even bottom line as a target for the
  1985 fiscal year, which necessitated a zero-based budget review of
  over 500 hospital cost centers
- The expedited opening of the newly constructed and renovated
  facilities to take advantage of the buildings' efficiencies of space
  and requisite service adjacencies

To successfully achieve these strategic goals and continue the turnaround, a major team effort was required. The team comprised not only hospital management and staff, key government officials, and bankers but also the board and Kinnard, who kept the hospital's vision in the forefront as tough operational decisions were made and implemented. The hospital's construction had to be kept on schedule, and its credibility had to be kept intact.

The 1985 budget process, commencing in the fall of 1984, proved to be an important vehicle around which change could take place. The zero-based budget review allowed senior management to examine every program, service, hospital cost, and potential source of revenue. 1985 was the year major sections of the new facility would open, so working capital in excess of $4 million provided by the FHA construction mortgage became available. This capital, combined with the correction and proper allocation of construction costs within the construction budget, gave the hospital a unique opportunity to creatively use the cash available to restructure its cash position. By April 1985, the $5 million line of credit and related interest expenses were eliminated. The austerity budget reflected two major efforts begun in late 1984 that were mentioned above: the closing of the Buffalo General Hospital School of Nursing and the elimination of acute care services at the Deaconess Hospital. Both carried a high risk of negative public relations, something the hospital did not need following a major nursing strike and during the clutter and dirt of new hospital construction. The media impact of the school's closing was initially significant; however, as the details of the closure were made known, this issue disappeared from media attention. The elimination of acute care services from Deaconess was far easier as the last acute care patient was moved from the facility in July 1985. Very positive media attention was gained as the transition took place, leaving Deaconess as a thriving skilled nursing facility with 108 beds. By 1987, it would have 162 beds. A moderate level of financial stability was being realized. All short-term debt had been eliminated. The financial plan was on track for the year, and the hospital had begun experiencing the efficiencies of the new building.

Along with the improved physical plant, environmental changes, and a growing sense of financial recovery, a recognizable improvement in morale was apparent. It was no more apparent than with the increasing support of the physicians and their use of the hospital. The construction program and Deaconess Hospital merger had, by the end of 1985, reduced the hospital's beds from 1,071 to 850. Yet with this decrease, three sectors of the physician staff grew in prominence, activity, and involvement with the hospital, as their morale and support of the organization improved.

Under a new SUNY@B faculty practice plan, the full-time faculty grew not only in numbers but in their responsibility for the clinical management of service programs throughout the hospital. Selective hospital investments were beginning to take form in orthopedics, cardiology, cardiac surgery, internal and family medicine, and physical and rehabilitative medicine. (These investments were made in accordance with the hospital's current strengths, opportunities identified as consistent with the BGH plan, and the planning needs of the Western New York community and within the role and function of the Buffalo General tertiary care mission.)

The private practicing physicians who had historically been the core of the physician staff not only continued to provide high-quality clinical care through the admission of over 85 percent of all patients but also carried a teaching responsibility for over 150 residents.

A new group of physicians arrived on the scene—physicians from Health Care Plan (HCP), a staff model HMO. By 1985, HCP had approximately 50,000 members. The hospital and HCP developed a contractual relationship under which, in return for an advantageous hospital rate structure, HCP would hospitalize its entire adult population at Buffalo General. A new and growing group of physicians, along with increasing HCP membership, provided an added volume of patients for the hospital.

Because of meeting the 1985 budget targets, the favorable changes in the hospital's cash position, and the improving relationship with the physicians, operational progress was being achieved. The bottom-line losses that had plagued the hospital during the previous four years had ceased by 1985, when a bottom-line gain of $235,000 was recorded. The operating loss had been narrowed from $4.8 million in 1984 to $1.4 million in 1985.

As financial stability became reality, so too did the desire and need to continually finance hospital program and service growth. By bringing Buffalo General's financial structure back in balance, the achievement of the vision remained the target. New hospital construction was fully completed by 1986, but renovation would continue through early 1988. The challenge was to sustain and repeat what had been achieved in 1985, to ensure that stability had taken hold. Nurturing the improvement was now all important.

The Hospital had achieved, in 12 short months, a significant change in financial position. Beyond these fundamental changes, other important infrastructure requirements were needed to complete the turnaround.

The information systems at Buffalo General had not kept pace with the changes taking place in the hospital industry. Financial instability and other hospital events did not allow for the planning, financing, and acquisition of a hospital-wide computer system. From an information perspective, the hospital was flying blind, not having the proper data to make important decisions. By 1986, it became imperative to replace the antiquated and limited financial information system and to install a comprehensive, flexible, hospital-wide information system.

An information systems leader was recruited, and a systems plan was completed. To maintain the hospital's fragile financial position, the prime emphasis of the first phase of the information systems effort was to immediately gain timely and accurate financial data. After selecting the SMS Independence System, the hospital once again called on Coopers & Lybrand for specific implementation planning assistance. In any financial systems conversion, the accounts receivable (AR) operations are the most vulnerable.

Because of the number of accounts, the value of those accounts, and the unreliability of the previous system, the hospital chose to have Coopers & Lybrand actively involved in all its business office operations through the AR conversion.

As a result of the involvement of Coopers & Lybrand and a strong hospital team effort, at no time during the conversion did the inpatient AR exceed 90 days. In addition, this effort, along with our financial management approach, improved our cash position from $164,900 at the end of 1984 to $9,723,000 at the end of 1988.

Since 1986, other major components of the system have been installed on time and with limited difficulty. As a result, new and more precise methods of communicating correct information have been achieved. The capture of all hospital charges and service visit and encounter data is nearing 100 percent. Major improvements in the hospital's operating room, nurse scheduling, laboratory order entry, and results reporting have been successfully implemented. The laboratory system has now been networked to HCP, as well as a 50-physician multispecialty group practice and a 7-member obstetrics and gynecology group, both at multiple sites.

A second major alteration to the hospital's infrastructure was to broaden its capability to respond to change. The highly restrictive regulatory environment that New York State is known for is no where as present as in the hospital industry. Although well intentioned, much of New York health care regulation is often so limiting that other less regulated techniques must be developed to maintain a competitive advantage.

It was in response to such regulation that the hospital extensively reviewed alternatives. As a result, it determined that a corporate restructuring of the hospital corporation was required to yield the necessary flexibility. A parent holding company model was created not only to hold Buffalo General but also to engage in other transactions that could be more easily developed outside Buffalo General with less regulation while still directed toward serving the broader interests of the hospital.

Among those programs and activities were the development or ownership of a nursing home, the imminent ownership of another hospital, four distinct types of home health care operations, a variety of physician-hospital joint ventures, and a property management and development company.

The hospital now operates as the flagship of the parent holding company, leveraging the strength of its improved acute care facilities and operations into a broadly based health care delivery system. The vision for a new Buffalo General has become reality, with a new vision for growth as a comprehensive health care system.

Conclusion

As with any evolutionary change, challenges remain that Buffalo General must face. In 1987 and 1988, the hospital continued to demonstrate the results of the financial gains made in previous years. Maintaining a positive operating margin in a federal and state environment that has placed New York hospitals last of all 50 states in comparative operating margins continues to be a challenge. With the eroding of hospital assets, hospitals in the state will be further behind in their ability to deliver leading edge medical care.

In addition, Buffalo General has continued to work on minimizing the amount of time patients stay in the acute care setting. The hospital diagnostic, therapeutic, and support systems have become interdependent. To optimize the quality of each patient care episode and to limit the cost of resources consumed, a constant and diligent effort is being focused on each element of the patient's stay.

To achieve an optimal stay, the hospital is continually challenged in its ability to accumulate, transfer, and analyze data for informed clinical care and the management of clinical and service outcomes. The goal is full hospital-wide automation in the early 1990s. The building blocks are in place, and the hospital is currently approaching decisions on leading edge technology for data transfer in key areas such as expert systems development, bedside monitoring, and clinical areas (e.g., radiology).

Another important area that deserves attention at Buffalo General is the institution's continuing contribution to graduate medical education (GME). Historically, it has been an important hospital mission, and in the foreseeable future it will continue to be. However, with changes in GME payments, the hospital, working with SUNY@B, will endeavor to make the university faculty practice plan nearly or completely self-supporting. This effort would limit the flow of hospital patient care dollars to the ever-increasing GME faculty costs.

Finally, the hospital must undergo another self-evaluation, perhaps more extensive than that done in 1985. A further test must be done on how far the hospital has moved in its constituents' eyes, since that is the only way it will truly know if it has made any difference over time and if the vision for the future is truly secure.

10

PRODUCT-LINE MARKETING TO INCREASE REVENUES IN A SMALL HOSPITAL

Jeanne Bouxsein Parham

Editors' Note: The uniqueness of this chapter is that most of its focus is on increasing revenues in a small hospital. The institution had a dramatic turn-around because of the numerous high-quality specialty programs it initiated to increase revenues. These programs, how they were initiated, and their effect are well documented. The emphasis on physicians and their importance to the turnaround of a hospital is also described throughout the chapter. The hospital was unique in both the number of specialty programs that it developed and the nature of these programs for such a small facility. It should be of value to anyone running a small to midsize hospital.

A hospital, with its peculiar dynamics of change and its mission of teaching and healing, has a life and personality that exists from the moment the doors open. The public knows this personality as the hospital's reputation; vendors and bankers assess its life by cash flow; but once given the opportunity to manage the rendering of care and services to the sick, one realizes a hospital has a life that must be nourished and a personality that can be shaped. So a brief history of the beginnings of Crawford Memorial Hospital in rural northwest Arkansas is necessary in understanding the events that lead to the period of decline in this hospital's life.

History

The opening of the 50-bed Crawford County Memorial Hospital in 1951 followed a three-year effort by a small group of visionary citizens of Van

Buren, the county seat. In 1948, their efforts culminated in voter approval of a $250,000 bond issue. The county court chose the Sisters of St. Benedictine the to operate the hospital under a lease agreement that called for a $1 a year payment. The original hospital staff consisted of 8 Benedictine nuns and 25 employees.

For years, the hospital thrived in this rural, farming community of 6,100. By 1968, the facility had been renovated twice and was competitive with the two hospitals across the Arkansas river in the twin city of Fort Smith.

In 1970, the construction of a three-story addition added 49 patient beds and modernized the clinical, diagnostic, and treatment capabilities of the hospital.

Falling Behind the Times

During the 1970s, the facility headed into its period of decline. Once able to compete with neighboring hospitals in terms of technology and services, the hospital languished as the Benedictine Order was unable to fund the technological advances that occurred in the 1970s. Local physician specialists elected to restrict their practices to the Fort Smith hospitals. Patient days were lost. Revenues declined, and the small physician primary care staff was demoralized.

Facing eroding public confidence, empty beds, and closed wings, the county's leaders decided to terminate the operating lease with the Benedictine Order. While the Sisters' ability to deliver compassionate care was undisputed, the officials knew that a change in management was necessary for the survival of the hospital and protection of the county's most valuable asset.

After a one-year period of being courted by various for-profit and not-for-profit suitors, the county entered into a 26-year operating lease in 1981 with a large proprietary chain. Their relative lack of experience in operating small, rural hospitals was overshadowed by their willingness to agree to a $775,000 annual lease payment. The prospect of doubling the county's general revenue fund also helped quell concerns raised over leasing the hospital to a for-profit organization. Their comfort level was improved by a lease covenant that called for the operator to provide an annual, preset dollar amount of charity care.

During the first five years of the lease, the operator was required to provide a $5 million equipment and physical plant renovation. Their strategic plan included recruiting speciality physicians from out of the area to service the hospital and its primary care staff. This plan backfired as it totally ignored long-standing referral patterns and further alienated the local specialists. The confidence of the citizens continued to erode with the hospital's inability to provide any specialty care.

After losses averaging $200,000 a month, the operator sold the operating lease in 1984 to a smaller proprietary chain from Dallas. At the time, this company had earned its reputation by performing financial turnarounds of unprofitable rural hospitals. With their strength in this niche and an orientation towards supporting local physicians, it seemed as if the hospital had found a good operator fit.

A new administrative team hired by the new operator charted a two-pronged survival plan of reducing operating expenses and rebuilding physician support. An unprofitable obstetrics service was closed and nearly 40 FTEs were laid off in the fall of 1984. Then, early in 1985, the hospital established the state's only cosmetic surgery program. While many scoffed at the idea of such a specialized program succeeding in rural Arkansas, they underestimated the primary strength of a marketing product line— participating physicians. So despite the devastation of employee morale by layoffs, wage freezes, and hours reductions and the straining of the public's confidence even further by the closing of the county's only obstetric service, the hospital became the first in the area to enter into product-line marketing, a bright spot that would become integral to the effort to revitalize Crawford County Memorial.

The hospital ended its first year of operation under the new operator with a loss of $570,273 on gross revenues of $6,481,498. Their average daily census for the fiscal year ending April 1985 was 24. When the administrator resigned, the associate administrator was appointed to that position in an attempt to provide some continuity in leadership.

A Turnaround Strategy Develops

The new administrator was faced with a pressing challenge: unless the hospital quickly adopted an aggressive turnaround strategy, the operator would walk away from the lease.

All turnarounds are underscored by hard work and patience. If they are designed to set the hospital on a course of long-term success, they also take time. Since most hospitals fail financially due to years of carefully cultivating a bad reputation, there is no magical way to restore financial health overnight. Under the new administrator, certain strategies were initiated that would move the hospital in the right direction although the hospital would continue to experience pretax losses through 1986. The strategies were interrelated and had to be implemented simultaneously to expedite the turnaround.

The strategies were:

- further strengthening physician support through the recruitment of established specialty physicians,
- identifying product-line niches in the market, and
- establishing a superior customer service program.

In May 1987 as these strategies were being put into place, the operating lease was again sold to an established, small operator of rural hospitals from Florida. The administrator was retained, and that year the payoff of the strategic plan was apparent in the bottom line. In 1987, the hospital had a $1.4 million operating profit on patient revenues of $13 million compared with a loss of $817,000 on patient revenues of $8.3 million in 1986. Average daily census had increased from 27 to 40 patients per day. In one year, the hospital made a 200 percent improvement in its pretax profit margin, from −10 percent to 10 percent, and for the first time in over ten years, the hospital was operating in the black. In 1988, the trend continued. The hospital posted a $1.9 million operating profit on revenues of $19 million and a census of 48 patients per day.

The Turnaround Approach

Communication was the first priority in developing the strategies for the turnaround. In 1985, the hospital's newly appointed administrator initiated weekly breakfast meetings with the medical staff to encourage their input and to keep the physicians informed of upcoming changes.

Employee meetings revealed a staff that was willing to work hard and go the extra mile given the opportunity to work for a leader with belief in the potential of the hospital. They were tired of hearing the line, "I wouldn't take my dog to that hospital," and wanted their day in the sun. They were confident in their care, and indeed, the quality of care rendered was the sole reason the small staff of primary care physicians had remained loyal during the hospital's bleak years.

The board of trustees was expanded to include voices representing the entire county. After assessing the hospital's strengths and weaknesses and listening to the concerns of the medical staff, board, and employees, the three-pronged strategic plan emerged.

But the plan needed time to have a fighting chance. What had came back to haunt the hospital's survival was the lease payment to the county. Though not due to begin until 1987, the facility was reserving for the future $775,000 annual expense. This reserve had a deleterious impact on the financial statements. The administration and board of trustees felt that the negotiation of more favorable lease terms would encourage the operator from Dallas to stay and support the turnaround plan.

In a long, exhausting year of meetings with county officials, a plan emerged that gave the hospital the expense reduction it needed to convince the operator to stay and seek success while assuring the county that, with the hospital's growth and success, they would see a commensurate return of the lease payment. The lease payment was reduced from a fixed annual payment of $775,000 to a $250,000 annual base lease payment plus one percent of annual gross revenues up to $10 million, two percent of annual gross revenues in excess of $10 million, and three percent of annual gross revenues in excess of $15 million.

The year's negotiations culminated in a meeting with the county court in a courtroom packed with hundreds of hospital supporters cheering on physician testimonials. Displaying the same fortitude that they had when the lease with the Benedictine Sisters was terminated, the court accepted the renegotiated lease payment plan. The court members fielded numerous complaints from citizens who failed to see the wisdom in giving anything back to the "out of towners in three-piece suits."

The lease payment reduction bought the time needed. The operator had a renewed commitment, and the county had a hospital. A strong message was sent throughout the area: Crawford County Memorial Hospital was not ready to give up. It had a personality to shape.

The Mighty Bridge

Crossing over the river was one of the hospital's biggest obstacles in recruiting local specialists. The bridge that connected Fort Smith and Van Buren appeared to have a concrete barricade on the Fort Smith side that kept specialists from performing work in Van Buren. Yet magically, the concrete barricade did not slow the migration of Crawford County residents to the two hospitals in Fort Smith. At this time, in 1985, the hospital's medical staff consisted of six primary care physicians. Every area specialist had offices in Fort Smith, near one of the two competitor hospitals. A chief complaint of Van Buren residents was having to travel to Fort Smith for anything serious. And, the primary doctors were unhappy over losing control of patients admitted to specialists at Fort Smith hospitals.

Almost exclusively, the recruitment of Fort Smith specialists to the hospital has been through the development of a product-line market niche. And the first market niche pursued at Crawford Memorial was cosmetic surgery.

Cosmetic surgery. In January 1985, a cosmetic surgery program entitled You're Becoming was launched. The only two board-certified plastic surgeons in the area joined the hospital's active medical staff to direct this program. It was a window of opportunity. There were no other cosmetic surgery programs within a 150-mile radius; the two physicians were highly respected and marketable; and both had dreamed of spending their last years of surgery practice performing elective cosmetic surgery. The start-up cost of the program was $250,000 for outfitting an operating suite and renovating private rooms and Van Buren office space.

The first week of advertising resulted in 250 inquiries. Since then, not only has this program gone on to become the premier cosmetic surgery program in Arkansas and Oklahoma, but it has generated incremental reconstructive procedures as well. Once the plastics surgeons had access to a surgery suite, they would add reconstructive cases to their cosmetic work to fill their schedule. In the first four years of this program, 582 cosmetic and 444 reconstructive procedures were performed at Crawford Memorial.

The You're Becoming program has evolved into the Arkansas Center for Plastic Surgery. This elevation reflects the program's success, experience, and recent accreditation by the American Association for Accreditation of Ambulatory Plastic Surgery Facilities.

In addition to the tangible benefits of increasing activity, the cosmetic surgery program paved the way for marketing other specialty product lines. The hospital had shown an ability to develop new business for specialists. It was the proving ground for programs to follow.

Cataract surgery. The Gift of Sight, a consumer-driven cataract surgery program, featured no out-of-pocket expense. Four ophthalmologists joined the medical staff and participated in this program. Cataract surgery was new business to the hospital. Eighteen procedures were performed in the first month of advertising. Until 1989, when the program was discontinued due to the government's reduction of outpatient surgery reimbursement, the hospital performed two hundred cataract procedures per year.

Impotency. In 1986, the hospital found a niche in impotency and developed Impotency Solutions. Several things lead to the belief that this program could be successful.

- Demographics. Arkansas has the second highest percentage of persons over the age of 65 in the United States.
- Renowned specialist. The urologist involved in the development of this program had been a leading penile implanter since 1977.
- Timing. Like cosmetic surgery, impotency was starting to come out of the closet. The year the hospital started the program, two major network news programs featured segments on impotency treatment, marking the first television coverage of the disorder.

In 1987, the program name was changed to the Southwest Impotency Center. The change reflected the leading position the program assumed in treating impotence in the southwest United States. Each year, urologists from all over the world and throughout the United States visit the Impotency Center. In the first year of operation, 710 inquiries were received, and 29 surgeries were performed, generating $173,907 in new revenues. Again, this product line not only generated implant surgery procedures but also led to increases in other urologic surgery due to the loyalty it created and the surgeon's preference for filling a surgery day.

In the three years of the program, 225 implants have been performed, generating $1,310,584 in gross revenues. Since the procedure is not on the Health Care Financing Administration's outpatient pricing list, it remains a profitable product line. Before this program began, the participating urologists generated $17,000 a month in hospital revenue. Through the program surgery and incremental surgery, these same surgeons now generate over $200,000 a month in revenue for the hospital. Additionally, they have relocated their practice from Fort Smith to Van Buren.

Same-day surgery. Crawford Memorial wanted to promote a service its competitors could not provide. An extension of the cosmetic surgery unit was developed for a same-day surgery unit featuring beautifully appointed private rooms, a complimentary meal for family, and a check-up call from the day surgery nurse following the patient's return to home. Once this campaign was positioned, the hospital advertised podiatry, gynecology, and knee surgery under the same-day program.

The growth of the hospital's outpatient surgery volume contributed significantly to increasing net revenue. The percentage of surgery cases referred through the same-day surgery product lines was, and remains today, a significant portion of its total surgery volume.

Prostate Center. The Southwest Prostate Center opened in April 1988. This product line was modeled after the Southwest Impotency Center and featured prostate ultrasound services for the early detection of prostate cancer. Crawford Memorial was the first health care entity in the area to offer this technology. During eight months of operation in that first year, 1,225 screenings were performed, with 90 surgeries performed for the treatment of prostate diseases.

Chronic Spine Pain. Perhaps one of the most important specialists missing from the hospital was orthopedics. A hospital that cannot set a broken bone is not people's first choice for cardiac care. The administrator had made several attempts to recruit orthopedic surgeons from Fort Smith. What was needed was a product line that would attract an entrepreneurial orthopedist. Chronic spine pain was a niche waiting to be developed. There were no providers in this heavily industrialized area offering holistic, multidisciplinary treatment for chronic back pain sufferers.

In one of the orthopedic groups the hospital had attempted to recruit, one orthopedist seemed ready to make a change. Strangled by his group's structure, this surgeon sought greener pastures in Van Buren. He was offered the medical director's role for both the chronic spine pain program and the hospitals orthopedic unit. This physician had one of the largest orthopedic practices in the area, and he specialized in back care.

The Chronic Spine Pain Unit opened in 1986. In the first six months of operation, the program generated $300,000 in new revenues. Like with the surgical product lines, new incremental orthopedic business added significant revenues as well. The chronic spine pain program has since evolved into an outpatient program, satisfying the insurance companies' need for cost-effective care. The hospital's agenda had been met. Orthopedics was a vital part of the facility's turnaround.

Attracting family physicians. In mid-1986, the administrator turned the recruitment efforts back to the hospital's bread and butter business: primary care. Again, the strategy to attract established physicians made sense. Established physicians would be less of a threat to the primary care physicians in the community, and an established physician would have a loyal patient following. An infusion of new family practice physicians would provide a stronger referral base for the growing specialty staff.

That year, relationship building commenced with two of the busiest family practitioners in the area—one in a small community 30 miles from Van Buren and the other across the river in Fort Smith. The approach taken with the physician practicing in Ozark, a community 30 miles from the hospital, involved repeated visits to her office. At the time she was the admitting physician for nearly all the patients in the Ozark hospital. This hospital was struggling under ineffective management, and the physician was discouraged by many instances of inferior quality of care. Early in 1987 after a year of courting, the physician transferred 22 patients in one day from Ozark to Crawford Memorial Hospital.

This physician continues to be a key admitter to the hospital and averages 60 admissions each month. Persistence and delivery on assurances about patient care and service, DRG management, and specialty support not only attracted the physician but have cemented this relationship. The hospital operates a courtesy transportation service between the two cities, minimizing the inconvenience of the 30-mile drive for the patients and their families.

In that same year, gynecology, neurosurgery, and general surgery practices from Fort Smith followed the lead of the plastic surgeons, ophthalmologists, urologist and orthopedic surgeon by opening full-time office practices in Van Buren. The active medical staff roster had increased threefold since 1984.

The gynecologist left a stifling multispecialty clinic practice for some newfound independence, and the neurosurgeons joined the staff to participate in the chronic spine pain program. They are an invaluable referral source for the orthopedist.

In early 1988, a Fort Smith family practitioner chose to leave his clinic affiliation of 11 years and set up an independent practice in Van Buren. The hospital provided a financial package that included an income guarantee, a no-interest lease on equipment and furnishing, and a loan that was used to resolve some personal debt. Today this physician is a leading primary care earner in the Fort Smith–Van Buren area and the hospital's second leading admitter. The hospital created the opportunity for his success, the culmination of over 18 months of ongoing dialogue, patience, and hard work.

Industrial medicine. Looking toward the future with a belief that the private sector will control health care costs in the 1990s, Crawford Memorial opened the Industrial Medicine Center of Northwest Arkansas in late 1988. Designed to help businesses contain health care costs through discounting strategies and health promotion programs, several of the established product lines fit with the objectives of the Industrial Medicine Center. The product lines and the physicians who had been recruited—orthopedists, neurosurgeons, plastic surgeons, urologists, and family practitioners—were integrated into the Industrial Medicine Center.

During the program's first year, 324 employee-clients were treated through the Industrial Medicine Center. In 1989, over 2,000 employee-clients have been treated. This increase is an obvious statement about the wisdom of choosing to target industry.

Quality of Care Strategy

Working hand in hand with the hospital's recruitment success and product-line marketing was a program that might be the unheralded source of the facility's turnaround. The hospital business is a tough business. A hospital services many demanding customers: patients, doctors, and payers. The administrator felt that the challenge in managing a health care system was in creating a process that offered the best possible outcome to the patient.

Customer service is now an industry buzzword. But at Crawford Memorial, quality of service became a focal point as early as 1986. Our program is not fluff. It's a way of life, and the attitudinal shift that must occur hospitalwide in a hospital oriented toward true guest relations and quality of service takes time to develop.

People pay a lot for hospital services. They expect value in comfort, convenience, rules bending, home-cooked food, warm blankets after surgery, and milk cartons that are easy to open. Patients deserve to understand their hospitalization. And they like knowing that the care provider still cares once they have gone home.

It was important to create a vision of customer service. The hospital managers were given the tools to innovate and continually improve the rendering of service. All staff pursued this mission by attending a guest relations training course called Memory Makers in a local luxury hotel known regionwide for its superior customer service. The ambience was exactly what the staff hoped to create in the hospital. Managers participated in the development of service indicators that were incorporated into the quality of care assurance program. Employees began to think beyond the constraining boundaries of a heavily regulated institution. Instead of *why?* they began asking *why not?*

At the top, administration had to make a commitment to live guest relations. Exceptional service deserves exceptional recognition, support, praise, celebration, and financial reward. To that end, the key management staff first addressed the environment they wanted to create for their employees. They wanted employees to care for patients. They felt it necessary to commit to some additional staffing, like a physician hostess and patient-family educators.

Value was placed on customer service through an extra-miler program. Each quarter many employees were recognized by their peers for going above and beyond the requirements of their jobs to assist a patient, family member, physician, or fellow employee. A member of the administration responded to each patient questionnaire. If a physician or patient complains, a satisfactory, lasting resolution becomes a priority. From the top on down, the focus is on the customer: patients, physicians, and employees.

That's why Crawford introduced a number of changes through the guest relations program. Ambience was important; a hospital does not have to look like a hospital, so rooms were softened. Other extra touches included gourmet meals, admission baskets, plush robes, free newspapers, and an afternoon courtesy cart with wine and cheese. Dress for success uniforms were provided for business office personnel.

Two popular components of the guest relations program have been extending the courtesy transportation service implemented to serve Ozark, and the HERO (Health, Education, Rural Outreach) Van. This self-contained vehicle travels to outlying areas in the county and performs free preventive care screenings for hypertension, cholesterol, diabetes, colon cancer, vision, and pulmonary function. The HERO Van has also become an integral part of the health promotion efforts of the Industrial Medicine Center.

To make sure the guest relations efforts work, quality service standards—like the temperature of a whirlpool, the wait for an x-ray, discharge instructions, hot coffee, and painless needle sticks—are tracked in each department. Quality of service is a way of life at Crawford. Customer service means repeat business, not just by the patient but by everyone the satisfied patient comes in contact with.

The hospital credits guest relations with the success achieved through word of mouth. Hospital care has so few tangible outcomes to which a patient can relate, superior customer service gives patients something concrete to share with neighbors and friends.

Telling the Public about It

As the hospital's competitors held their breaths wondering what new product line the facility would introduce next, the hospital embarked on an image campaign to let the public know how the hospital had changed.

"Better than ever" was the theme that was promoted in a series of high-touch television commercials and newspaper advertisements that centered on patient experiences with the hospital. The campaign highlighted four years of hard work in achieving its day in the sun. Crawford Memorial, today a 103-bed facility, is now positioned as an alternative to the large hospitals in that it offers comparable technology and facilities and a level of customer service unmatched by any.

Looking Back

While several million dollars have been spent adding state of the art equipment to the hospital over the past few years, this equipment would sit idle without the support of a growing multispecialty medical staff. Only physicians order the diagnostic services and treatments that generate revenue for hospitals. For a rural hospital competing with nearby tertiary care centers to survive and prosper, it was essential to establish the primary care and specialty physician base necessary to offer full medical and surgical services to the community.

The strategic plan of recruiting established physicians, developing product-line niches, and incorporating a strong sense of customer service into every task performed was focused and driven by many individuals who became shareholders in the process. The hospital has entered a new era and has no time to rest on its laurels. Operating in the dynamic field of health care and from a position of financial prosperity, the strategy will now change.

The reward of this turnaround has been more than financial. It has opened the door to new opportunities for many employees. It has given the physicians and staff the opportunity to perform their best work with a full array of technological support in an ambience of pride and enthusiasm. And this hospital, now nourished, is headed for a long and successful life.

11

THE TURNAROUND IMPERATIVE: FROM VISION TO RESULTS

Richard J. Frenchie

Editors' Note: This chapter describes the turnaround of a midsize hospital. It provides a broad description of the strategic actions that were needed to bring the operation from a deficit to a financially sound position. Special emphasis is placed on the programs that were expanded and the programs that were discontinued. In addition, the interaction with the medical staff and the importance of physician recruitment is discussed. Then the marketing and communications initiative and its importance to the turnaround are reviewed. Lastly, a brief overview of the strategic planning process that was used is provided in the exhibits.

Corporations can generally be divided into two distinct categories: reactive and proactive. When confronted with adversity, a reactive corporation buries its head and hopes the problem goes away. A proactive corporation, on the other hand, digs in its heels and meets the challenge with decisive aggressiveness. Additionally, this fervor and intensity transcends the entire corporation from top to bottom.

Geauga Hospital was confronted with adversity in 1988 with respect to its short- and long-term fiscal viability. Its leadership was faced with two choices: Be reactive and risk the very survival of an essential health care facility, or be proactive and attack the problem honestly and aggressively. At that critical time, the hospital made a bold decision to adopt an organizational model that would be patient driven. The model emphasized the need to look inward and examine all hospital operations. Proactively, internal changes were orchestrated to develop a vision for the future. The hospital identified the challenge—to improve quality and productivity at a competitive price—and met that challenge by implementing innovative strategies.

The drive to succeed engaged everyone at Geauga Hospital from top to bottom. Consequently, adversity motivated the hospital to define its strategic direction and unite to move toward a position of strength in the health care marketplace. This thrust paralleled the contemporary thinking of Leland Kaiser, a health care futurist, when he urged, "Health care must be redesigned to be patient centered. The hospital should be a healing community. Hospitalization should be a guided experience to heal, transform, renew, empower and involve the patient."[1]

What follows in this chapter describes the forces that molded one community hospital's strategic vision, and details a kaleidoscope of events that made its vision a realization.

Preturnaround Profile

Geauga Hospital is a 169-bed, full-service, community hospital near Cleveland, Ohio. It is the sole acute care hospital in Geauga County, and its relevant market (area closest to the hospital) embraces a population of 100,000 of which the hospital currently receives a 38 percent market share. Situated in the center of a quasi-suburban-rural market area, the population profile ranges from the upwardly mobile, sophisticated, urban transplant to the educated conservative blue-collar worker to farmers, including a strong and conservative Amish element.

From the late 1950s through the mid-1980s, the hospital enjoyed program growth and development. This growth reinforced a sense of confidence and conservativeness. Moreover, as the sole provider in the county, there was a strong perception of security predicated on community acceptance and support. However, the mid-1980s brought a new wave of competitive threats, which, in part, eroded the hospital's market and financial strength. These outside environmental stresses heightened the need for the hospital's leadership profile to move toward a proactive role.

Table 11.1 clearly shows Geauga Hospital's financial trends over the last three years before the turnaround, revealing its vulnerable position. The difference between 1986 and 1988—$1,218,919—graphically demonstrates the sharp erosion of hospital revenue. The acceleration of losses for a community-based hospital without other major sources of revenue to draw on was an alarming trend. Major pressures that contributed to this condition were a lack of new physicians being attracted to the community, the encroachment of outside health care providers, the shrinking reim-

Table 11.1 Financial Performance Trends: Excess Revenue over Expenses

1986	1987	1988
$520,809	$109,354	($698,110)

bursement from payers, a highly leveraged debt position, declining utilization, and a diminishing market share.

To rectify major space and operational deficiencies, a comprehensive construction and renovation project was completed in mid-1987. The hospital's operating space capacity was nearly doubled, and state-of-the-art technology and advanced community and specialty services were added. The public's perception was changed by constructing a more contemporary and aesthetically pleasing physical structure. Yet, it was abundantly clear that bricks and mortar could not ensure future viability.

With the announced retirement in 1987 of the CEO of the past 20 years, the growing imperative for change began to take form with an eight-month search for a replacement. Governing boards in today's American hospital industry frequently look to the outside for top leadership talent. Geauga Hospital was no exception. The talents of the then executive vice president were considered, along with those of other top candidates, in an effort to find the leader best suited for Geauga Hospital.

Ultimately, the decision was made to appoint the executive vice president, whose association with the hospital spanned 14 years. The governing board clearly recognized that his detailed knowledge about the hospital and its unique problems would allow more rapid assessment and the adroit visionary management of existing operational and strategic issues. Moreover, the new CEO was under immediate pressure to demonstrate positive results within a very short time period. His ability to size up accurately the condition of the hospital; to communicate clearly to the governing board; and to move forward with a sense of continuity, aggressiveness, and a proactive vision created the chemistry for future positive changes.

Simultaneously, three major leadership positions within the hospital hierarchy changed hands: the CEO, the chairperson of the governing board, and the chief of the medical staff. The triad of new leadership powers now demanded a galvanized relationship with intense cooperation.

The leadership style of the CEO set the tone that built relationships within which issues were addressed honestly and directly. Since they were all new to their positions, the CEO was able to enhance the efforts of the three leaders beyond the conservative framework. The chairperson of the governing board was infused with new spirit and energy and a certain willingness to take risks. He brought an innate philosophy that through a collaborative spirit problems could be viewed as opportunities. The chairperson embodied much of Tom Peters' philosophy stated in *Thriving on Chaos:* "There are no excellent companies. The old saying, 'If it ain't broke, don't fix it,' needs revision. I propose: 'If it ain't broke, you just haven't looked hard enough.' Fix it anyway."[2]

Similarly, the chief of the medical staff moved beyond the traditional role in his commitment to quality and excellence. Thus a dynamic environment was created where new insight and a proactive commitment could immediately encompass the hospital leadership.

Postturnaround Profile

During the first three years of the turnaround, Geauga Hospital improved its financial performance from a deficit of $698,110 in 1988, to a net gain of $435,970 in 1991, as shown in Table 11.2. Given the limits on fiscal resources, the positive swing of $1,134,080 was a meaningful achievement in three years.

The most salient of the financial factors in the two-year turnaround from deficit to profitability are summarized below. The implementation of each initiative is explained in more detail later in this chapter.

- Increased new admissions by 300, which represented $1.5 million in new gross revenues
- Recruited 31 new practicing physicians in strategic community locations
- Instituted a new physician referral and hospital information service to direct new county residents to appropriate physicians or hospital medical services
- Developed direct contract (preferred provider) agreements with five local business establishments
- Expanded operating revenue through a revenue enhancement program, resulting in $1.5 million in new reimbursement
- Instituted self-funded health care insurance for hospital employees, reducing costs from traditional insurance premiums by 50 percent
- Assumed administrative and funding responsibility for the Workers Compensation Program, which reduced expenses by $80,000 annually
- Launch a self-funded professional liability insurance initiative, with anticipated cost savings of $150,000 annually

Table 11.2   Postturnaround Financial Performance: Excess Revenue
over Expenses

1988	1989	1990	1991
($698,110)	$14,043	$108,834	$435,970

- Reduced human resources by 16 FTEs
- Refinanced a revenue bond issue, which saved $2.5 million over the life of the issue
- Discontinued an unprofitable chemical dependency unit, reducing hospital expenditures by $350,000 annually
- Instituted a house physician charge system, generating $100,000 annually to help defray the cost of underwriting the service
- Initiated an ongoing, multifaceted, fund development program, a hospital first, which generated $333,000 in nonoperating income
- Enhanced hospital auxiliary efforts to develop new and unique fund-raising efforts, netting $63,000
- Developed proprietary ventures to further the health mission and contribute to the hospital's overall financial margin
- Instituted a product standardization and evaluation system, which reduced materials expenses by $50,000

A major marketing communications initiative was set into motion by the creation of a new marketing position successfully headed by a seasoned professional. The implementation of aggressive, upbeat, quality-oriented marketing communication programs were targeted to heighten awareness of the hospital and enhance its image. These pursuits contributed directly and indirectly in the turnaround success.

The creation of a new health care network also was an integral part of the turnaround profile. Simultaneous with the implementation of internal initiatives, Geauga Hospital codeveloped a formal network affiliation with a major academic medical center, University Hospitals of Cleveland. Six hospitals are currently members of the network. The affiliation did not result in a merger or the exchange of any material assets or liabilities but rather focused on opportunities to increase each member's effectiveness. Each member hospital made long-term commitments corporately approved by their respective boards of directors. An exchange of two board member positions by each hospital with University Hospitals formalized the affiliation, sending a clear signal of commitment. The membership work together in synergy to nurture the network and strengthen each organization's respective missions.

The linkage created the opportunity to provide a continuum of health care services, as well as potential satellite services from the main campus of University Hospitals to Geauga Hospital. A representative sampling of how this association has matured over the last few years shows the positive benefits and the real necessity for the hospital to affiliate with a network:

- Developed a joint oncology program
- Granted faculty positions for Geauga physicians in a major teaching hospital
- Facilitated the recruitment of physicians
- Developed a network-wide preferred provider organization (PPO)
- Created medical, administrative, and board councils to further develop network strategies
- Obtained a nursing grant of $500,000 dedicated to innovative patient care procedures (a sole community hospital generally would not be eligible for such a grant)
- Instituted a health information and physician referral system
- Designed medical consensus panels for clinical case management

The network association also vaulted Geauga Hospital into a new sphere regarding its image and presence in the community through the prestige associated with a major academic medical center. Modern trends were clear indicators that networking was a necessity for future viability.

The proactive, strategic thrust that propelled Geauga Hospital forward hinged on the consensus of the governing board, the medical staff, the administration, and management. A shared vision of a new future direction enabled hospital leadership to set goals that could turn around negative trends and sustain forward movement.

Finding the Pathway to Turnaround

The strategic planning process was the single most important organizational endeavor that lead to short- and long-term viability. The ability to communicate a new vision and to motivate the initial involvement of the governing board, the administration, the medical staff, management, auxiliary groups, and the community were all important in building a consensus with a sense of ownership. They were a part of the solution in the vision of success.

Under the leadership of the CEO, a fast-track strategic planning methodology was designed to take on a greater dimension than previous planning pursuits. It emphasized involvement and ownership at all organizational levels. The planning initiative was spearheaded by the CEO, who provided the planning groups with expertise while saving time and economic resources, as opposed to using an outside consulting group.

The strategic process involved a nine-phase approach, as enumerated in Exhibits 11.1 and 11.2. The first five phases consisted of a comprehensive assessment, which served as the nuts and bolts of the entire strategic planning effort. The process determined what the reality was and what the hospital could be in the future.

With the completion of the strategic planning environmental assessment data base, the next key phase assembled the leadership of the board, the medical staff, the administration, and management through a two-day Futures planning retreat. The retreat addressed three key tasks:

1. Assess the hospital's current position and the major forces that would affect its future
2. Given the forces at work, determine the outlook for the next three years
3. Determine what strategic initiatives were necessary to secure the future

Evolving from intensive discussions of the hospital's problems, the unanimous conclusion reached at the retreat was that three key issues needed to be addressed:

1. Utilization
   • Patient activity declining with shrinkage in market share
   • Increasing competitive threats
2. Hospital image
   • High patient satisfaction by users of the hospital
   • Significant competitor preference given the lack of hospital image and awareness
3. Financial
   • High cost per case
   • Highly leveraged
   • Growing net operating loss
   • Major reductions from third-party payers

Exhibit 11.1   Strategic Planning Process (Geauga Hospital)

  I. Develop environmental assessment data base

    A. Internal

        1. Admissions and days of care for 1985–1988 (projected) by
           a. clinical service or product line
           b. intensity/complexity
           c. age, sex. religion, etc.
           d. financial class
           e. referral source

        2. Utilization for 1985–1988 (projected) of
           a. beds by service or product line
           b. key hospital ancillary and support services

        3. Patient origin trends for primary and secondary markets by clinical service or product line for 1985–1988 (projected)

        4. Market share for 1986 and 1987 for primary and secondary markets by clinical service or product line

        5. Hospital financial trends for 1985–1988 (projected)

        6. Profitability analysis of clinical services for 1987 and 1988 (projected)

        7. Physician age and admissions analysis by clinical service or product lines for 1985 and 1988 (projected)

        8. Referrals to tertiary facilities by clinical service or product line for 1985–1988 (projected)

        9. Satellite activity analysis for 1984–1988 (projected)

      10. Inventory of programs and services by disease and key publics.

    B. External

        1. Trends in local residential and commercial economic development, including a brief regional overview

Continued

Exhibit 11.1   Continued

2. Trends in population (age, sex, income, religion, etc.) for 1980, 1987, and 1992

3. Overview of Medicare, Medicaid, commercial and Blue Cross and Blue Shield reimbursement initiatives

4. Key competitor utilization, market share, and financial trends, including program plans and cost comparisons for 1984–1987

5. Trends in physician supply and location for 1985 and 1987

6. Knowledge, attitudes, and awareness of key publics (consumer, physician, employer, etc.)

7. Trends in medical technology development

II.   Assess resources and program portfolio

III.   Conduct interviews to develop working hypothesis
   A. Medical staff
   B. Board of trustees
   C. Management
   D. Community

IV.   Conduct independent market research study

V.   Develop trends and conclusions from data base and research

VI.   Reassess hospital mission and develop strategic initiatives (planning retreat)

VII.   Develop strategic objectives

VIII. Establish implementation strategies and action plans

IX.   Implement action plans

The consensus of the hospital leadership was that an aggressive strategy was essential to ensure both short- and long-term viability. Consequently, based on these conclusions, the hospital adopted a strategic position that embodied a proactive vision to guide it through survival during the 1990s. The shared vision was simple, but compelling: Geauga

Exhibit 11.2 Geauga Hospital Strategic Planning Time Line (1988–1989)

Key Task	July	August	September	October	November	December	January
Environmental assessment							
Assessment of resources and program portfolio							
Assessment of health care market							
Interviews to develop working hypothesis							
Independent market research study							
Development of trends and conclusions from data base and research							
Reassessment of hospital mission; development of strategic initiatives (planning retreat)							
Development of strategic objectives							
Implementation of strategies and action plans							
Implementation of action plans							

Hospital must be the hospital of choice for patients and physicians in its relevant market area.

This single sentence provided a focus for all who shared in the planning for the future. The goals were realistically defined in such a manner that has kept the hospital focused on implementing the turnaround imperative. Implicit in the vision statement was the importance of excellence, punctuated with flexibility and adaptability to move the hospital into the future.

Tom Peters, in his book, *Thriving on Chaos*, alluded to this contemporary view of corporate vision when he said, "Merely aspiring to be excellent will prove disastrous; the only winning companies will be constantly adapting ones—organizations that are able not only to respond quickly to shifting circumstances, but to proactively take advantage of them, continually creating new market niches and adding new value (quality) to their products and services in response to the ever shifting desires of their customers."[3]

As the retreat approached closure, there emerged a clear consensus that three decisive strategic goals had to be pursued within the next three years to achieve long-term viability (see Exhibit 11.3).

1. To increase the utilization of Geauga Hospital and its medical staff
2. To deliver high-quality health care applying effective cost-management measures
3. To develop other sources of revenue through fund development and endowment programs

From Vision to Reality

Strategic goals were now clarified and the vehicles that would transform the shared vision into reality were initiated. Three task force committees were established, each assigned one of the three strategic goals. Each was composed of an equal number of board, medical staff, and administrative and management participants. The committees were directed to develop strategic action plans and define how the action plans were to be implemented.

The CEO opened the channel of communication, set the pace and the constraints, and acted as the catalyst for the whole planning effort. After the two-day retreat, the success of the planning initiative hinged on his

Exhibit 11.3   Geauga Hospital Strategic Vision and Goal Statements
                  (1989–1991)

Shared Vision

Geauga Hospital is to be the hospital of choice for the physicians and patients in its service area.

Goal I: Increased Patient Volume

By 1992

*   To increase patient admissions by 1,000
*   To increase the percentage of local residents (within defined service areas) using Geauga Hospital's medical staff
*   To increase the awareness of Geauga Hospital and its medical staff's capabilities
*   To develop a plan to utilize excess hospital bed capacity through differentiated services and programs

Goal II: Expense Control

By 1992 to initiate expense reduction measures without adversely impacting quality

Goal III: Nonoperating Revenue Generation

By 1992

*   To increase nonoperating revenue by establishing an endowment program and foundation
*   To develop health-related profit-making ventures through the hospital profit subsidiary

---

ability to communicate. He accomplished this task of clearly articulating the problems addressed during the retreat through personal and written presentations to the medical staff, hospital employees (by means of small group meetings), volunteers and auxiliary, the business community, and friends at large of the hospital.

Very briefly, his summarized message candidly stated, first, that the hospital's basic mission to provide quality care had not changed; second, that to solve the problems facing Geauga Hospital, new strategies were needed to accomplish the turnaround imperative; and, third, the specific actions required to achieve the strategic goals.

The CEO initiated three constraints integral to the achievement of the strategic goals, which the governing board, medical staff, and management leaders agreed to: (1) positive results toward a turnaround had to be effected within two years; (2) layoffs or major work force reductions would not occur; and (3) hospital rates would not be increased.

Major Initiatives Influencing the Turnaround

The task force committees functioned as autonomous units, but they did not work in isolation. In fact, the committee members developed dynamic interactions with input flowing freely among committees, peer groups within the hospital, and the community at large.

The most influential actions affecting the turnaround were driven by three specific strategic goals that emerged from the planning process. The three task forces developed these actions, while the CEO assumed their implementation to ensure a continued high level of motivation and ownership throughout the hospital. The significant actions implemented to fulfill the three strategic imperatives are summarized to provide a perspective on the significant financial impact.

Heightened Utilization

In the first year of the turnaround, patient care activity increased by 300 inpatient admissions as compared to 1988. The major contributing factors in this positive achievement were physician recruitment and medical staff development, marketing and communications, and revenue enhancement measures.

Active physician recruitment increased the medical staff by 31 physicians. The recruitment process was guided by a well-designed policy and plan with the complete input and support of the medical staff, board of trustees, and representatives of the community. The plan articulated physician need by specialty as well as the designated geographic areas underserved. The recruitment sources consisted of networking with medical schools, residency programs, established physician practices, search agencies, other physician networks, and the University Hospitals Network. The plan further provided the necessary financial support and incentives to attract practitioners to associate with the hospital.

The marketing and communications initiative focused on raising the awareness of the residents in the hospital's service area about the hospital and its medical staff. Beginning with the recruitment of a top-notch and resourceful marketing and communications professional, a carefully designed plan identified measures to achieve this fundamental purpose. Among the multiple elements of the plan, the most salient include the following:

- Physician promotion in the various print media resulted in extensive visibility and attention for the hospital and its spectrum of services.
- A community newsletter brought information on contemporary health issues and available hospital programs to the service area and differentiated the hospital from competing health care facilities.
- Community outreach programs exhibited health services of the hospital and medical staff at local malls and public facilities to provide health prevention information and beneficial health screenings. Community outreach pursuits included services such as diabetic, cholesterol, and colorectal screening services; smoking cessation programs; cardiac and stroke rehabilitation clubs; cancer support groups; and numerous educational forums and seminars.
- A high-profile, multipurpose awareness publication featuring the hospital's vision and new directions created increased interest and dialogue within the community.
- A thematic series of visible advertisements, emphasizing the hospital's uniqueness, strengths, and capabilities, were developed, wrapped around a comprehensive media campaign.
- The instituted physician referral and hospital information services drew the community to the hospital and its medical staff by developing new relationships.

The inception of direct preferred provider contracts with five area business firms, spearheaded by the CEO had an immediate impact on patient volume increases. The objective of these preferred contracts was to develop a committed patient volume while assuring quality and affordable health care for the business community close to home.

Expense Control

Three self-funded, hospital insurance programs resulted in a combined expected savings of $230,000 annually. Before these programs were initiated, extensive research was done to ensure that the expected cost benefits would be achieved through a good plan design.

Outside consultants analyzed the hospital's loss experience for professional liability over a ten-year period revealing the clear economic advantage to self-insure through the creation of an insurance trust; savings were anticipated to be as high as $150,000 annually.

The self-funded health care insurance program for hospital employees ensured the hospital would be the preferred provider. Through the involvement of the medical staff in the plan design, the hospital enjoyed nearly 100 percent participation from both physicians and employees. The net effect resulted in a 50 percent decrease of annual employee health care expense increases compared to using an outside insurance provider. A self-funded workers' compensation program was the third segment and demonstrated a cost savings potential of $80,000 per year.

Another cost-containment initiative reduced human resources. With a commitment to reduce staff without layoffs, several positive techniques were implemented. Cross-training within departments made staff more flexible. Attrition reduced the staff some. Employees were allowed excused absences without compensation when the workload decreased. A temporary hospital-based staffing pool was used to acquire human resources when patient volume spiked. Flexible staffing involved extended 10- and 12-hour days and varying shift times. An early retirement program was also initiated. All these measures have been successful and generally accepted because employees were aware that they had to be a part of the solution in reducing hospital expense. Involvement and communication were the keys to success.

The implementation of a hospitalwide productivity system resulted in a 98 percent measured efficiency rating. Management monitored work load and work force requirements and thus amended procedures and systems to manage fluctuating activity and acuity.

Expense controls were further enhanced with the refinancing of a revenue bond issue, which saved more than $2.5 million over the life of the issue. By taking timely advantage of lower interest rates, about $100,000 per year was saved.

The hospital discontinued its unprofitable chemical dependency unit in 1990. After five years of aggressive market development and promotion, the service continued to drain resources from general operations. The annual savings amounted to $350,000.

A reexamination of house physician services, a program provided at no charge to the patient or the physician, has resulted in cost reductions.

A change in policy to permit the hospital to selectively charge for emergency medical procedures, histories and physicals, preadmission testing procedures, and other services rendered by the house physicians provided $100,000 in annual reimbursement to help defray the cost of underwriting this program. The medical staff was involved in the policy revision to avoid any conflict in hospital charges versus physician professional fees.

An extensive audit of the hospital pricing structure and charge system revealed that revenue from a significant portion of reimbursable, billable services was being lost. A decision was made to revise the information system and capture the chargeable services. This initiative enhanced revenue by $1.5 million without adversely affecting the hospital's competitive stance in the health care marketplace.

Nonoperating Revenue Generation

The ongoing fund development program was instituted with a clear set of the program's objectives and action initiatives. The objective was to build an ongoing endowment fund of $10 million in ten years. A fund development committee, including board members, medical staff leadership, and community representatives, was charged with the responsibility to reach out to potential community leaders to seek their financial support through contributions and fund endowments. The CEO, without the use of additional staff, assumed the administration of the fund development initiative. Operating expenses were minimal as measured against the return of $333,000 in funds generated.

Fund development was a first for Geauga Hospital. Several facets of the fund initiative include an annual campaign to reach the community at large and local businesses, special gifts, endowments, select foundations, and special events.

The effort to generate new revenues also involved the hospital auxiliary. In the past, the auxiliary had been the major fund-raising group; now they were being challenged to reach out more innovatively than ever before. This involvement was achieved through new events such as golf tournaments, a Night at the Races, jewelry and shoe sale bazaars, fashion shows, and fine art shows and sales. The auxiliary's varied efforts to raise funds represented a multifaceted program and dedicated community volunteers. Their efforts raised $63,000.

The development and enhancement of proprietary ventures also added a meaningful contribution to the overall margin during 1989 and 1990.

Suburban Health Care Management Services, Inc., is a wholly-owned, for-profit subsidiary corporation of Geauga Hospital. Created in 1985, its principal mission is the provision of service-oriented ventures in health care. Revenues generated from the subsidiary are exclusively used to further the health care mission of its parent, Geauga Hospital.

The subsidiary corporation consists of four ventures: Culinary Design Catering Service, Evercare Home Emergency Response System, Home Infusion Therapy Care, and a durable medical supply equipment company. The home infusion service and the durable medical equipment services were added since 1988 and provide a continuum of health services consistent with the hospital's strategic vision.

The subsidiary's consolidated financial statements for 1990 revealed a 113 percent increase in net income over 1989, based on total gross revenue of $187,609.

External Forces Impacting Turnaround

Geauga Hospital's turnaround centered heavily on the internal actions specified above. This internal strategy was necessary to meet the immediate challenge of creating a positive change in the hospital's financial operations. It is important to note that while some outside influences at times adversely affected the turnaround efforts (for example, fiscal restraints by government payers and intensified competition), others were beneficial. A selective sample of such influences are summarized below.

Government Affairs

The turnaround benefited from the input of two individuals: a member of the board who served as an Ohio state representative, and an Ohio state senator who was a long-time resident of Geauga County. They supported the new hospital vision and pledged to influence, through the political process, issues and health care policies affecting hospitals in general, including Geauga. The state senator was most helpful in challenging several insurance carriers regarding reimbursement to the hospital and aided in reversing several denials.

Patient and Community Support

As the community's knowledge and awareness of the hospital's new vision and defined pathways expanded, significant levels of support and affirmation were realized. In fact, civic and community service groups as well as businesses pledged their strong support and participation in several strategic initiatives, particularly those involving physician recruitment, fund development, and new services in conjunction with the University Hospitals Network.

In addition, through patient tracking systems, the hospital received high marks, as reflected in a 95 percent and higher patient satisfaction level. Such responses focused on existing services and initiatives implemented as a part of the turnaround. This data clearly communicates patient and community support.

Marketing Communication

The inception of a marketing communication plan created new opportunities to expose the public to the hospital. Increased media coverage boosted the community's awareness of the hospital and its services. The University Hospitals Network connection provided increased marketing capabilities, such as exposure in a four-color glossy network consumer magazine. This enhanced visibility and image awareness.

Third-Party Payers

Through the hospital's selective and highly aggressive negotiations from a position of strength with third-party payers, more favorable reimbursement rates were realized.

The Future

The direction for the next two years (1990 and 1991) will be aimed at sustaining current momentum and building on the success achieved thus far. By continuing to carry out the actions outlined in the strategic plan and by setting attainable goals that reflect that plan, the hospital will use its previous successes as building blocks for the future.

At the onset of the hospital turnaround, a $2.5 million improvement in fiscal operations over a three-year period was unanimously considered doable. In 1989 and 1990, the hospital fulfilled a significant portion of this goal. To fulfill the vision of long-term viability, the right moves already in place must continue in tandem with new actions for 1991 and 1992. Such actions include the following:

- The hospital needs to find specific program and service niches that more clearly differentiate it from its competition and design persuasive marketing tools to fill those niches.
- Ongoing fund development is essential for the hospital to reach out to the community and be proactive with its fund-raising efforts.
- A patient quality service initiative will focus on patient sensitivity and expectations.
- The affiliation of a tertiary care facility through the University Hospitals Network should be used for image building and the development of new or enhanced services such as the strengthening of the obstetrical services by the creation of a neonatal unit, the recruitment of a neonatologist and high profile female obstetricians, the recruitment of a critical care specialist, and clinical expansion of the critical care unit.
- The hospital must identify and implement the best option among the following for utilizing bed capacity: a subacute care unit, a respite care center, a geriatric and psychiatric center, and an ambulatory care center.
- The hospital must institute an employee incentive program and profit sharing program.
- The hospital must institute cost management measures, such as selective contracting for clinical or nonclinical services and the development of hospital-based radiology and emergency physician groups.
- The hospital must continue to promote the its new identity and image and enhance the existing physician referral and health information service.

A Look Back

Rarely does one find leaders of institutions that have dramatically changed who would not change a single decision, no matter how small. Geauga Hospital was no exception. However, the hospital's leadership does not regret any decision made during the turnaround. If they had to do it over again, they would follow the same formula.

In retrospect, the following are among the hospital's best actions taken during the turnaround:

- The creation of a winning organizational spirit
- A commitment to building and nurturing internal hospital relationships
- A commitment to quality and excellence with adaptability
- A disciplined approach to strategic planning that addressed the present reality and a rational approach to determine the course to ensure present and future viability
- Linkage with a tertiary academic medical center to synergistically provide a continuum of health care services

Actions that might have enhanced the turnaround include

- more aggressive interaction and participation in the political process and government affairs, and
- a greater consensus between the hospital and medical staff regarding the delivery of health care services (i.e., hospital-based services versus physician office–based services), the development of alliances and partnerships with the medical staff, and a better definition of its role in relationship to the hospital.

Conclusion

It is clear that Geauga Hospital has set the course for continued viability. The record of achievements in two years bodes well for the carefully constructed three-year vision. The transition to a highly proactive, winning-spirit philosophy created enthusiasm for both the hospital and community.

In the next few years, the hospital must chart its course in the health care waters amidst uncertainty and mounting pressures. Industry issues will focus on quality and cost management. The Geauga Hospital course must include the continued expansion of quality patient care, the institution of new cost-control measures, and the shaping of services and programs that are consistent with its community health care mission. Aggressive marketing will promote the vision to be the hospital of choice for the community. Coupled with these initiatives, continued fund development efforts will provide the economic resources to pursue the established pathway.

One common thread runs through the Geauga Hospital success story: its people. Over the rich 32-year history of the hospital, numerous adversities and challenges have assailed it. In each case, dedicated staff have risen to the challenges and ultimately created a better and more efficient operation. The hospital's key philosophy that its human resources hold the key to success is clearly manifested throughout the organizational fabric. Successful organizations do not achieve success by accident; resourceful employees make it possible. With renewed spirit and a commitment to continuous quality, Geauga's staff augers well for the patient and community alike.

Notes

1. L. Kaiser, "Visionary Governance," (Presentation at the Health Trustee Institute, Cleveland, Ohio, March 5, 1991).
2. T. Peters, *Thriving on Chaos: Facing Up to the Need for Revolution* (New York: Knopf, 1987), p. 3.
3. Ibid., front jacket.

12

TURNAROUNDS: AN EPILOGUE

Terence F. Moore and Earl A. Simendinger

Turnarounds, whether of institutions of 42 beds or 1,042 beds, appear to have a broad range of factors in common even though they might take somewhat different approaches depending on the character of their boards and administrations and the size of the institution. In smaller institutions, the CEO is more directly involved in all aspects of the turnaround; in larger institutions, the CEO is no less pivotal to the turnaround's success, but the top management team implements most of the turnaround strategies. Effective chief executives of medium or large hospitals and health care systems have learned what good military commanders have known for centuries: a general's job is not to fight; a general's job is to build an army and lead it.

Signs of Organizational Decline

The most tangible sign of organizational decline is a worsening financial situation. The financial standing of the organization finally reaches an unacceptable level that demands administrative changes (this level is sometimes above a break-even level but most often is below a break-even level).

Other characteristics are also common to almost all hospitals where the gap between potential performance and actual performance is widening. First, in such an organization there is an inordinate amount of bickering; conflict seems to be the norm rather than the exception. Bickering is frequent and open. Formal committee meetings erupt into damning remarks about the way the organization is being operated.

Secondly, issues are not resolved on a timely basis, consequently, these unresolved conflicts eat at the organization like a cancer. Months and even years pass, and the same battles are being fought—sometimes by the same players. The situation is analogous to watching a soap opera and then turning on the television a year later and feeling one has not missed a thing. The same players are acting out the same counterproductive roles.

Third, there is a sense of resignation. Employees, like a beaten army, are resigned to an ignominious fate.

> Nowhere is this more clear than at the middle management level, where employees feel as if they are sitting in a traffic jam waiting for a broken red light to change. Only the top level managers present a front of optimism, but even they occasionally show the physical and psychological effects of being resigned to what they consider "fate." These administrators may remind keen observers of an aged elk or deer that is at bay and about to be brought down through repeated attacks by a pack of wolves or of a prizefighter who is physically and emotionally spent in the later rounds of a fight, but whose legs will not buckle under his opponent's punches.
>
> A sense of resignation may arise under several circumstances. For example, an administrator who was told he had only two more years to serve as the chief executive officer of a 350-bed hospital before he would be placed on a consulting status went into a two-year "glide pattern." He was verbally attacked both by the medical staff and by the administrative staff. Because the board of directors did not name a successor, the hospital lost two years in terms of its development; the present administration is scrambling to catch up.
>
> Another administrator who was in his early sixties hinted to his hospital's board of directors that he would accept an early retirement if the package were liberal; however, he retained as much decision-making power as he could. The board did not have the wisdom to remove the administrator from the organization, and the cost to the organization in lost opportunities was far in excess of what it would have been to pay him even his total salary to retirement age without working. [1]

Fourth, there is stagnation in the way the organization views opportunities and addresses problems. There is stagnation in the way employees are treated and a tendency to justify what is being done because it worked in the 1970s.

Lastly, there is a lack of vision about what the organization should do not only to respond to the environment but also to influence it. Management spends more time responding to the latest crisis rather than developing an agreed on intermediate and long-range plan.

Michael Rindler is more emphatic and states that a yes to any one of the following questions means that a hospital should be turned around:

1. Has the hospital operated at an operational loss for two or more consecutive years?
2. Are activity trends significantly worse than those in competing hospitals?
3. Are trustees holding private meetings to discuss "concerns" or hiring outside management consultants to evaluate the CEO's performance?
4. Has market share declined for two or more consecutive years?
5. Is the hospital always responding to marketing initiatives of competing hospitals, rather than the other way around?
6. Are physicians controlling policy decisions because of a weak board and management?
7. Are competing hospitals or a hospital chain offering to buy or merge with the hospital?
8. Are the hospital's bankers expressing concern about the ability to cover fixed expenses like interest on outstanding loans?[2]

Stages of a Turnaround

G. Robert Durham, CEO of Phelps Dodge Corporation, outlines four stages of turnarounds.[3] They are as follows:

1. Evaluate your assets, people, and facilities.
2. Identify your strengths and weaknesses.
3. Agree on realistic, attainable goals. Divide these goals into specific tasks to be achieved by specific members by a certain time.
4. Hold progress meetings monthly.

Although there are numerous typologies for the various stages of a turnaround, perhaps the best analysis comes from John Gabarro.[4] Gabarro believes that most stages of a turnaround could be defined as either learning or action. The five specific stages that he outlined are (1) taking hold, (2) emerging, (3) reshaping, (4) consolidation, and (5) refinement. These stages appear to be consistent with the process outlined in the various chapters of this book. The only major difference is that hospital turnarounds appear to occur in shorter timeframes than those described by Gabarro.

In the taking hold stage, there is much learning and action. Perhaps the best terms to describe it are orientation and evaluation. The CEO is becoming oriented to the environment and evaluating both the people and the programs. Most of the changes that take place during this stage are corrective and affect areas that need immediate attention. This first stage ends when the situation appears to be fairly well understood.

In the emergence stage, the manager immerses himself or herself in running the organization in a more formalized fashion. Fewer changes are made during this phase, and it is a period of temporary stability. This second stage ends when the management develops a more detailed concept of how to improve performance and how the organizational structure should be altered.

The reshaping stage is the period of most intense change. In this stage, the manager acts on the learning of the previous stages and begins to act on it. Most structural changes in the first three years of a turnaround are made during this stage. Often, it can include significant reorganization and downsizing. We have seen this stage take place as late as a year into the turnaround process and as early as 30 days after a new CEO has arrived.

In the consolidation stage, Gabarro states that "The manager and his group attempt to consolidate the changes made during the reshaping stage. The learning early in this stage tends to be evaluative, focusing mainly on the results of the major changes made in the early period."[5]

The refinement stage is the last stage and is characterized by the manager's additional learning as a consequence of day-to-day problems or running the business rather than a need to work on major problems. This is the fine tuning of the organization. The CEO coming into a well-run organization might find himself or herself in the refinement stage and have the luxury of not having to go through the other phases. One program popular in hospitals during the past few years that is characteristic of the refinement stage has been quality improvement programs. These programs are designed to develop a formalized methodology for employees to be involved in decision making and problem solving. Hospitals all across the United States are spending hundreds of thousands of dollars to develop such programs, which use a distinct methodology to enable work teams to analyze and solve problems. These programs are a tool to help sustain a turnaround.

Another program that is standard to many hospitals is a suggestion program. One of the most successful suggestion programs in the United States is at MidColumbia Medical Center in Oregon. The program has a hospitalwide focus that begins with the orientation program. The CEO places great emphasis on this program and personally reviews all suggestions. One of the unique features of the program is that the suggestions are not only for cost savings but for improving services. Quarterly, the employee with the best suggestion is awarded a weekend vacation in a resort area where the employee and his or her family are taken by limousine. The impressive result of the program is the more than 100 suggestions per week the CEO receives from approximately 450 employees. In some major health care institutions in the United States, the CEO has weeks in which he or she does not receive a single suggestion for improving the organization's operations from anyone but his or her spouse.

Gabarro describes his various stages as the three wave phenomenon. There are definitely three waves of activity accompanied by lulls in the activity. There is a period of relatively high activity during the initial taking hold stage. Then the activity levels drop off but reaches its peak during the third or reshaping stage. During the consolidation stage, the level of activity again drops off, but some additional activity takes place during the refinement stage.[6]

For our purposes, we broadly define the stages of a turnaround as the diagnostic phase and the revenue increase and expense reduction phase. Of course, follow-through needs to be ongoing because a successful turnaround is a continuous process, not an occurrence that only takes place in a finite period of time.

The Diagnostic Phase

The diagnostic phase can begin even before a CEO arrives at an organization. Tim Stack, CEO of Borgess Hospital, wisely suggests that a CEO who accepts a position in a hospital that needs turning around should begin the diagnostic process before he or she arrives. Exhibit 1.1 shows a suggested list of the materials that the CEO should review before and after arrival. Conducting such a review in the initial stages of the diagnostic phase can save considerable time, and this familiarization with the organization can enhance the gathering of additional information because the CEO is better prepared to ask the right questions of the right individuals.

A review of the minutes to many key board meetings before arrival can provide the CEO with a grasp of what has happened and the positions various board members have taken. The longer board members have been on the board, the greater the likelihood they feel the hospital is their own and the more they tend to want to be involved in operations. This principle is particularly true of board chairpersons who have held that position for a long time (five years or longer). It might also be true that a board chairperson's willingness to delegate responsibilities for the operations to a CEO are inversely proportional to the amount of time the board chairperson has been in office. A board chairperson who has been in his or her position for ten years is less apt to provide sufficient latitude to the CEO to conduct a turnaround than one who has only been in office for a year or two.

Most CEOs have found that the diagnostic phase of the turnaround can best be conducted by holding a large number of one-on-one interviews with people, both internally and externally.

Some CEOs have focused their attention on people outside the management team to determine how they perceive the situation. Thomas Rockers, former CEO of Santa Rosa Medical Center, stated that he decided to block out any opinions of the present management staff and discern how physicians, both those utilizing the facilities and how those who did not utilize the facilities, as well as board members, viewed the situation. He reported the process took six months. This investigation was done concurrently with interviews of several business people in the community each day in which Rockers asked them the following questions:

1. Tell me how you think Santa Rosa Healthcare Corporation can better serve the community?
2. What did we do wrong?
3. What did we do right?
4. How can we improve?
5. Will you help me?

Joe Smith, while president of Gladwin Area Hospital, implemented a comprehensive survey that each department manager completed. It assessed service delivery, consumer satisfaction, supply consumption, staff utilization, market potential, program effectiveness, and interdepartmental systems. From this analysis, a list of operations improvement objectives was formulated. Such a survey, in addition to providing a great deal of information in a short period of time, also serves two other functions: (1) It forces the individual department managers to evaluate their operations (that should be their job anyway). (2) It can highlight the ability of the various departmental managers to complete an assignment, measure their writing skills, and see how they follow through on diagnostic abilities.

Daniel Rissing, CEO of St. Raphael Hospital, New Haven, Connecticut, also believes in the importance of one-on-one meetings with employees to determine what should be done. He began a long series of one-on-one sessions with board members, the top 25 medical staff admitters, and every middle and top manager. Wisely, he noted that most of the conversations were one-way—the physicians did most of the talking.

Gary Goldstick states that a turnaround manager (of any company) must determine the answers to the following ten important questions:

1. What is the stage of adversity?
2. What is the status of the present and near-term cash position of the company?
3. What are the critical issues that need to be addressed immediately in order to ensure the continuation of the business?
4. What is the liquidating value of the balance sheet? [This question might not be of great importance to the health care executive.]
5. To what extent is the firm exposed to secured creditors (both short-term and long-term)?
6. What are the objectives of the board and other principals?
7. What is the recent historical performance of the company?
8. What is the realistic forecast for the company's profitability and cash flow?
9. Are there potential product breakthroughs or immediate "miracles"?
10. What is the status of the basic business elements?
    a. Is there a viable core business in the company?
    b. Are the employees skilled and loyal?
    c. Is the middle management competent and loyal?
    d. Are the owners [board] cooperative and committed? [7]

Regardless of how the diagnostic phase is conducted, it must be thorough because it serves as a basis for the actions that will be taken if the turnaround is to succeed. If false conclusions are drawn, they will result in false starts—something many hospitals in need of a turnaround cannot survive. In this stage, listening is the chief communication skill, and it is clear that the CEO and the top management must listen to a number of publics, including the board, the medical staff, employees, and community leaders.

Revenue Increase and Expense Reduction Phase

Once the diagnostic phase is complete and financial targets have been determined, the revenue increase and expense reduction phase begins. The meat of any successful turnaround is the actual steps taken to reduce service expenses and increase revenues. This phase is multifaceted because so many areas are affected.

Communications. Communication is so important during the revenue increase and expense reduction phase that it merits some additional attention. A CEO's ability to communicate during a turnaround can be the most critical aspect of his or her success. A CEO who cannot communicate effectively cannot lead. Moreover, there is no substitute for direct verbal communication between the CEO and all supervisors as well as with the employees at all levels.

Stewart makes some suggestions about how an executive should conduct himself or herself when communicating the turnaround strategy.[8] First, be personal; shake hands and call employees by their first names. Second, establish some optimism even though the situation might appear to be grim at the present time. Executives should tell employees that they have confidence in the employees' ability to effectively execute any plan that is approved at the board level. Third, encourage teamwork. Remind them that no one should take glee that someone else is a part of the boat that is sinking. Remind them that all are in the same boat and teamwork will shorten the time it takes to turn the organization around.

Finally, show that the executives have a grasp of detail. Do not try to influence them with a series of cute sayings and platitudes. Show them that the executive is personally aware of the situation by presenting a strategic overview of the organization's position and why it is in its current state. If the meeting is with a particular department, be well versed in that department's operation before addressing the group. Ask for an additional detailed briefing from the department supervisor if necessary. In addition, be gracious and be sure to thank the employees for their time. Also take this opportunity to comment on future communications and encourage the employees to contact their respective supervisors with any questions at any time.

One last rule of thumb in a turnaround is information is like fertilizer and should be broadcast throughout the organization at every level.

> A good turnaround manager is able to transmit energy quite far down the organization. He must have the leadership skills that are required to revitalize the company, and he must communicate that he does possess these skills. He must be able to clearly state the mission of the organization, communicate that mission, articulate how all shareholders will benefit from achieving that mission, and express confidence that success is possible. He must imbue employees with a sense that the situation has changed, the company is now on course, and something is going to happen shortly.[9]

Revenue increase. The techniques health care executives employ to increase revenues might often be directed toward longer-term results, but efforts to initiate them must begin as soon as possible.

One strategy is to build on existing service lines. If the hospital has a large group of orthopedists, it might be advantageous to build a sports and fitness operation or add a psychiatrist and develop a rehabilitation unit.

Another strategy is to develop totally new service lines. The recruitment of select specialties and the development of new medical service lines were dramatically highlighted in the chapter about Crawford Memorial Hospital by Jeanne Parham. Even though Crawford Hospital was small, it developed a cosmetic surgery program and gave it a catchy title, You're Becoming. The program then did 582 cosmetic and 444 plastic reconstruction procedures in its first four years.

The cosmetic surgery program was followed by a cataract surgery program, which now performs between 20 and 40 surgeries per month at Crawford Hospital. Other successful programs at Crawford are impotency clinics, same-day surgery, a prostate center, and a chronic spine pain clinic. The administrative team also recruited much needed family practitioners and established an industrial medicine center that has been a resounding success. This type of development and expansion of medical services can do as much as anything else to increase a hospital's revenue.

Some health care executives have turned their hospitals around almost solely by recruiting much needed physicians. An outside consulting group, such as Oberfest, that can assist in developing a comprehensive physician staff plan is recommended to provide some objectivity and credibility and to take some of the onus off the management team.

Another strategy is to develop a comprehensive but focused marketing program. This is discussed further under the section on the role of marketing and public relations below.

One final strategy to increase revenues is to increase select charges. Even in an environment of Medicare and Medicaid reimbursement, this strategy can often produce additional revenue. Some hospitals, in an attempt to be the lowest-cost hospital in the area, have reduced their capital reserves to such a low level that they will never be able to catch up with their competitors. Again, outside consultants can be invaluable in analyzing and determining where charges could and should be increased. Often they will work for a small percentage of the revenues they actually generate.

Staff reductions. Since 55 to 60 percent of the costs in most hospitals are salaries and benefits, reductions in the work force are usually a high priority strategy in a turnaround. Hospitals that have been turned around often have a lower percentage of salaries and benefits. Archbishop Bergan Mercy Hospital's salary and benefit costs, as a percentage of total revenue, went from 48.5 percent in 1986 to 36.3 percent in 1989.

The popular term for reducing staffing levels is downsizing. Downsizing can be done without outside assistance, but it is often done with the expertise of one of the major health care consulting firms such as Friedlander and Kachmarik describe in Chapter 9.

Rindler outlines several questions that must be asked to guide the direction of the downsizing of the hospital's staff.

1. Should the hospital use layoffs or hour reductions?
2. Should it reduce salaries instead of laying people off?
3. Should it use seniority or competence in layoff decisions?
4. Will bumping be allowed?[10]

Most of the authors selected the payout strategy rather than the salary reductions, but sometimes both techniques must be employed. However, there is a limit to how few employees an organization must have to provide quality service. If the number of employees is reduced to an intolerable level, even basic tasks cannot be performed. That situation occurred when Joe Smith cut the staff of the Gladwin Area Hospital from 134 FTEs to 109 FTEs. These cutbacks did not enable the hospital to reach a break-even point; therefore, all employees were forced to take a 16.4 percent wage decrease or the hospital would close.

Some suggestions from those who have successfully instituted this phase of a turnaround: First, the worst day of the week to announce a layoff is Friday, because it gives the employees all weekend to react without having any supervisors around. Second, the CEO and top executives should not be perceived as receiving increases or new perks such as leased cars during this time. The management of General Motors lost considerable credibility several years ago when, in the middle of severe cutbacks, it awarded large bonuses to most of its top executives.

Third, the need to treat those who are being laid off with care and dignity cannot be overemphasized. Progressive hospitals use outplacement firms and provide other assistance to help minimize the trauma associated with layoffs. One COO who was terminated during a recent downsizing said the most important thing he learned in the entire process was that he would never terminate a competent manager without giving him or her the opportunity to first find another position. It is far more difficult for someone to find a position when they are unemployed than when they are employed because of the stigma associated with being unemployed. Clearly, CEOs do not often have the luxury of giving their staff the time to find other positions before being terminated. Nonetheless, some of the greatest atrocities being committed to health care professionals today are by their fellow health care professionals during attempted turnarounds.

Reduction of services. Sometimes the reduction of select staff is not enough, and entire services must be reduced or closed. This was the scenario at Ancilla Systems when it divested itself of St. Anne's West, a 50-bed facility in a northwest suburb of Chicago.

The increasing emphasis on service line management and the information provided by DRGs enable most hospitals to determine which services are money makers and which services are losers. Although a hospital must often provide a full range of medical services (both winners and losers), it should most often place greater resources on the more profitable service lines.

In determining which services to reduce or eliminate, the Society for Healthcare Planning and Marketing has offered the guidelines listed in Exhibit 12.1.

If eight or more responses support reinvesting, the organization should continue with the program or service. If eight or more support divesting, serious consideration should be given to closing or selling the service. If the answers are evenly divided, the service should be modified.

Supply reduction. Supply expenses account for between 15 and 25 percent of the total operating expenses of a hospital depending on the classification and overhead expenses associated with the purchase, distribution, and storage of supplies. Supply expenses are second only to salaries in total hospital expenses and can be a rich source of saving.

Finding savings in the supply area is similar to searching for truffles, a mushroom-like plant that grows below ground and is considered a great delicacy by many. The areas where significant savings can be made are often not readily apparent, but they are there. The following are some areas to look for savings in supplies:

Exhibit 12.1   Guidelines to Eliminate Services

	Reinvest	*Divest*
Were the actual financial results anticipated in the business plan?	Yes	No
Has the business been operating less than 18 months?	Yes	No
Is there at least one example of a known profitable operation of about the same size of your planned operation?	Yes	No
If utilization targets have not been achieved, what is the reason?	We have not achieved but still think it is reasonable to do so.	Overestimated demand.
Is your payer mix the same as or better than you expected?	Yes	No
Is this a high fixed-cost operation?	Yes, we could increase utilization without adding expense.	No, expanding services means adding expenses.
Can you quantify spin-off benefits to the system?	Yes	No
Can you identify any real competitive advantages you have in the marketplace?	Yes	No, we're about the same as our competition.
Can you identify specific management actions that can reverse the losses?	Yes	No
Is this a mature product or line of business?	No	Yes
Would you use your own money to invest in this venture.	Yes	No

Source: J. Green, "Which Services to Reduce," *Modern Healthcare*, August 18, 1989, p. 29. Reprinted with permission from MODERN HEALTHCARE. Copyright Crain Communications, Inc., 740 N. Rush Street, Chicago, IL 60611.

- Food is a major expense, and studies should be conducted to determine if the cost per meal is competitive with other hospitals of a similar size. Is the cafeteria operating at a break-even level and is catering being abused at meetings and conferences?
- What is the turnover rate of replacing linens, and are permanent press items being used optimally? Along with these questions, an analysis of the cost per pound of doing laundry should be conducted.
- Money can be saved on x-ray film if contracts have not been negotiated recently.
- Disposables account for a major expense in many hospitals. Is it less expensive to use disposable dishes than china? Has such an analysis been completed recently?
- Maintenance contracts might not be considered as a supply expense, but they can be a source of cost savings. One hospital with a $90 million annual operating budget had $1 million in service contracts.
- Stockless or just-in-time inventory, product consignment, and product standardization can reduce supply expenses.
- Medication and intravenous (IV) solutions are often considered a supply expense, but they are so important they should be considered separately. Perhaps the greatest potential for savings in a pharmacy lies in the establishment of a formulary that restricts the number and types of drugs being used in the facility. This issue can be very political and should be developed and adjudicated in the pharmacy and therapeutics committee. The inventory in a pharmacy can be measured by its turnover. A pharmacy that has an annual turnover rate of 15 is probably operating at near perfection. A turnover rate of 5 is not uncommon, but indicates that the pharmacy inventory is too large. Finally, IV contracts should be evaluated to determine if they are competitive.
- Utilities are probably overrated as a source for savings. The use of computerized heating and air conditioning systems that control room temperatures when the rooms are in use or not in use have saved significant dollars, and most hospitals should have them, but simply turning lights out in hallways and other areas will probably result in insignificant savings.
- Dues and subscriptions are another area where waste is often found. The hospital should examine its relationship with professional

associations and also ensure that the duplication of subscriptions is minimized. In one hospital, 32 top executives subscribed to the same magazine—all were paid for by the hospital.

- Design problems are sometimes the cause of space not being used productively. Just as most hospitals are not organized to do what they must do (many would argue that most were never organized to do what they must do), their structure often does not maximize efficiency.

   Excessive operating space can be expensive to maintain because of housekeeping, maintenance, and utility expenses. One hospital that successfully turned around its operations determined that "It had almost 1,100 square feet per bed, and hospital architects now suggest approximately 800 square feet per bed. In addition, the hospital had too many beds. Although 45 beds would have been more than sufficient inasmuch as peak patient load was 40 and average daily census was only 25, the hospital had 72 beds."[11]

   In this era of greatly reduced inpatient volume, many hospitals have excess capacity that translates into inefficiently used space. The reconfiguration of space to better fit the needs of various services and therefore the entire organization takes time but is often a worthwhile investment.

The reduction and elimination of staff and services necessitates a well-thought out plan and execution that is as flawless as possible. The CEO who focuses only on increasing revenues or only on downsizing gains half a loaf; both activities are necessary if a turnaround is to be successful.

The Role of Various Publics

The Role of the Management Team and Employees

The role of the employees has been described in every chapter and does not need further discussion.

One important duty of any new manager, especially in a turnaround, is to reduce the amount of sniff time with their employees. The term *sniff time* derives its origins from the time two dogs spend sniffing each other when they first meet. It is the time when the employees are determining what the new manager is like and learning about his or her expectations.

The best way to reduce the amount of sniff time for employees is for the manager to give a speech about his or her likes and dislikes. It might include such statements as the following:

- I like employees who are highly disciplined and demanding of themselves.
- I like responsiveness.
- I like people who follow up.
- I like clean work areas and good housekeeping.
- I do not like people who hide things.
- I do not like long reports.
- I do not like people who do not work as part of a team.
- I do not like people who speak poorly about their organization outside of work.

It is important that the sniff time speech be totally consistent with the manager's own performance standards. In other words, if the manager states that he or she likes employees who are open and available, then the manager should also have an open door policy and be available.

The importance of the management team cannot be overemphasized. Management teams are built on similar values, compatible expectations, and mutual respect.

One of the most important lessons to be learned from studying turnarounds is the importance of the relationship of the CEO to his or her managers. Gabarro states that "Perhaps the most salient difference between the successful and failed transitions was the quality of a new manager's working relationships at the end of his first year."[12] Every attempt must be made to cultivate an effective working relationship among members of the management team.

One additional phenomenon appears from our analysis of turnarounds regarding the CEO and his or her managers. In failed turnarounds, the CEO fires several managers soon after arriving (which is also true of successful turnarounds). The difference is when the CEO fires people he or she has hired after 12 to 24 months. The CEO then becomes a bull's eye for the medical staff, employees, and the board, and his or her position is overrun. For any CEO who is in the process of terminating many of the managers he or she has hired, the chances are great that the CEO will not have a long tenure.

Finally, it is interesting to note how few managers generally remain in a hospital after the five stages of a turnaround are complete. Some are fired, some leave, and some retire. Based on our observations, however, it seems that, on average, only one third are still working in the hospital at the end of the turnaround.

The Role of the Board

The role of the governing board in a turnaround is almost self-explanatory: to govern the actions of the CEO and the top management team.

The CEOs from the various chapters in this book who have successfully conducted turnarounds have all somehow managed to attain and maintain the support of their respective boards throughout the entire process. There are probably numerous CEOs who have lost their jobs attempting turnarounds because they lost the support of their boards along the way.

It should be noted that many boards have been an integral part of an organization's decline into financial difficulties even though they do not often receive the blame for it. Another factor at work in many turnarounds is that although the CEO is new, the board members have been in power for some time. Their loyalties to each other are often much greater than to the CEO they have hired to increase the financial standing of the organization.

Wise CEOs quickly discern the attitudes of the individual board members and if they err, they err on the side of overcommunicating with them. Key decisions, such as layoffs, the revision of long-standing policies, and decisions that are politically sensitive in the community and among the medical staff are all reviewed with key board members in advance to obtain their support. To do otherwise is to ask to have the limb one has gone out on sawed off behind one.

In summary, the role of the board is to (1) set policy; (2) review and, if approved, support the major actions of the CEO; (3) allow the CEO to represent it with the medical staff; (4) be available; and (5) increase its expectations of the CEO and management team, not its involvement.

Effective executives do not make the mistake of communicating only to the chairman of the board. The executive committee of the board or a select group of board members should be given the authority to approve, on a timely basis, major actions of the administrative team. Even the best CEOs often find themselves continually compromising between doing what they know should be done and doing only that which is politically acceptable.

Obtaining the support of the board throughout the turnaround is no less important than obtaining the support of the employees throughout the organization.

Mark Celmer, CEO of DeGraff Memorial Hospital, cautions that a CEO should be sensitive to the fact that prior decisions of the board were probably prudent ones at the time. Managing change is a matter of finesse, and the CEO should not alienate board members who feel or perhaps felt at one time that their important decisions were good and in the best interests of the hospital. Celmer says the successful CEO is one who can find a way to revise prior decisions of the board as necessary yet allow the board to retain pride of authorship in those decisions.

The Role of Planning

Some authorities believe that the development of a long-range plan is a luxury that, in a true turnaround, is not economical and that the organization does not have the time for. Survival becomes the overriding short-term goal.

If there is little consensus among the board, the administration, and the medical staff about where the hospital should be going, the development of a long-range plan becomes significant. In addition, if the board is prone to not condoning administrative initiatives unless they have been thoroughly analyzed and discussed, then a long-range plan can be invaluable in fostering consensus. Of course, the other major advantage of a comprehensive long-range plan is that it prioritizes what must be done and, if used properly, often saves considerable resources.

We strongly believe that a long-range plan should at least be done concurrently with the other turnaround efforts. If it is not, the organization will lose precious time when the immediate crisis passes.

The Role of Marketing and Public Relations

Both marketing and public relations play an important part in most turnarounds. The activities within this category are as diverse as they are numerous. Most are intended to enhance the hospital's image and improve the revenue side of the turnaround equation. Some of the more common activities conducted by our turnaround artists are the following:

- Special reports to the community enable the hospital to tell its side of the story and develop community support. These reports are most often published in the local newspapers, but they are sometimes mailed separately to all households in a community or region.

- Hospital open houses can be an effective public relations tool. These are usually well attended, especially if they are combined with free screening clinics.
- A speakers bureau made up of various members of the hospital's medical staff and health care professionals can help make the hospital more visible and reach key groups.
- Physician directories can be tailored to referring physicians or the general public. It is important that these directories be developed in concert with the medical staff.
- A packet of materials can be sent to all new members of the community shortly after they arrive. The packet contains a full array of information regarding the hospital.
- Special events such as hospital week, love light tree lightings, and the observance of other special dates and anniversaries can give the hospital a high profile.

Any type of marketing program should be based on sound marketing research. If adequate research has not been done, it should be done during the diagnostic phase of the turnaround. An added value of such research is that it can be used in a year or two to determine if community perceptions have changed as progress is made. Good market research can provide a level of credibility and clarity that is necessary to convince board members and members of the medical staff of how the organization is perceived. Executives do not suffer because they cannot solve their problems; they suffer because they cannot see their problems. Good market research helps identify real problems.

Most of our turnaround artists emphasize the importance of reviewing any major advertising with their boards, employees, and some members of the medical staff before it appears in the news media. Advertising can have a positive effect on the morale of employees, especially if the hospital has been receiving considerably less attention in the news media than its competition. Later, management might wish to focus advertising on select service lines. William Nicely and Joan Neuhaus note that they reduced marketing expenses from $800,000 in 1985 to $200,000 in 1988.

Employees can be a hospital's biggest public relations tool during a turnaround, or they can be its biggest problem. In a small- to midsized community, an uninformed and disgruntled employee work force can totally negate any other attempts to create a positive image for the hospital.

Richard Roodman and Cheryl Minckler of Valley Medical Center devote most of their comments (see Chapter 2) to outlining the importance of marketing in a turnaround situation. No organization appears to have spent more time and effort on developing an understanding on the part of their employees, managers, board members, medical staff, and others about what the hospital stands for. Like other organizations, they published a mission statement; but unlike other organizations, they developed a 36-page facts pamphlet that is distributed to all the hospital's internal publics. They offered a $50 dinner for two as a prize to anyone from these publics who took the facts quiz and passed it.

They report that the results of this annual program have been outstanding and unprecedented. Each year over 2,000 people are exposed to what Valley Medical Center is all about. Their employees have the opportunity and incentive to learn more about their hospital and, in turn, promote those facts to their customers.

The Role of Volunteers

Volunteers can be vital in a hospital turnaround. Their importance is often a function of how actively they are involved in the organization and how well they influence the key decision makers in the community. One small hospital described in this book had more than 100 volunteers who were active and also influential in the community. These volunteers played an important role in gaining community support and public relations during the downsizing of the organization. It is important that the volunteers be organized and active and that the administration communicate with them as it would with an employee throughout the process.

Michael Rindler took a gutsy step in his turnaround and actually terminated some volunteers who were working at the front desk of his organization.[13] These volunteers were not consistent or did not provide good quality service. Although it was warranted in his situation, it is probably the exception to how volunteers should be treated during a turnaround.

The Role of Consultants

Consultants have been used in about 50 percent of the turnarounds that we have studied. Consultants can save time and provide expertise and credibility. They are also expensive and therefore are not used in some turnarounds where they could be used.

In using consultants, it is important that they be used on projects for which in-house expertise is lacking and that they be directed by the administration. Occasionally, consultants report to the board and create more organizational friction than organizational improvement.

The Role of Physicians

With the possible exception of the board, no group can have a greater positive or negative effect on a CEO's ability to manage a hospital's turnaround than the medical staff. Without at least the passive approval of the medical staff, a turnaround is doomed.

The medical staff must be well informed of the turnaround plan, and their input into the plan must be sought. Even when they are well informed, they tend to be more concerned with the immediate effects any cutbacks might have on their own nursing units or other services rather than the hospital's long-term viability.

Mark Celmer, CEO of DeGraff Memorial Hospital, recognizes that most medical staffs attempt to adhere to the status quo. The only person who likes change is a wet baby. However, he believes that the ultimate success of the CEO in earning the respect of the medical staff is a function of the CEO's ability to turn every decision into a unified win-win opportunity. An organizational philosophy should strive for a win-win-win opportunity, placing the benefits to the patient and community first, followed by the organization and the physicians.

Sometimes many members of the medical staff believe that the hospital's losses are the result of accounting capers. Some will never be convinced that the hospital does not have sufficient income to cover its operations until the facility is forced to close.

If relatively inexpensive physician amenities can be developed, then they should be. Physician parking, physician dining areas, and other physician services can help foster an atmosphere that management is concerned with their welfare. Sometimes simple acts such as providing more accurate and timely reports can create a favorable impression on the part of many physicians.

In addition to keeping physicians informed and involved in the turnaround, health care executives should initiate the development of a physician staffing plan or a revision of the existing plan if a plan is already in place. Moreover, this action should be taken in the initial phase of the turnaround. The analysis of the type and number of physicians needed is part of the diagnostic phase of the turnaround, but it is so important it should be treated as a separate subsection of the diagnostic phase.

Physicians, like board members, are sometimes a major factor in the hospital being in an unfavorable financial position even though they might not overtly share in the blame for the unfortunate financial situation. Their reluctance to change, to thwart the recruitment of much needed staff, and their desire to keep things the way they are might have contributed more to the hospital's unfortunate position than any previous action by the administrative staff.

A physician staff plan can be developed without an external consultant, but the medical staff might perceive such a consultant as more objective. In addition, a good consultant will outline the number of physicians needed in the future to obtain targeted market share levels in most specialties. The board and the administration should make the plan with input from the medical staff. The medical staff only acts in an advisory capacity to avoid antitrust issues.

David Hunter, president of Hunter Associates of Chicago and one of the foremost experts on hospital turnarounds in the United States, believes that having a physician ad hoc advisory committee is key to a successful hospital turnaround.[14] The advisory committee provides advice on (1) managed care negotiations, (2) physician recruitment, (3) nursing improvements, (4) physician admitting patterns, and (5) physician service improvements.

This group of physicians does not interfere with the duties of the medical executive committee. However, it is prudent to include the chief of the medical staff as a member of this committee as a liaison with the formal medical staff committee structure. A side benefit is that physician members become more educated about the problems facing the hospital in a turnaround.

It sometimes becomes apparent that, regardless of a CEO's best efforts, a group of physicians is so entrenched in maintaining the status quo that they will not actively support administrative or even board decisions. In this situation, the CEO should consider the tactic most military commanders would employ: bypass them. Work around these holdouts. Work with other physicians if possible. If, for example, oncology, neurosciences, and obstetrics and gynecology appear to be services that can be expanded greatly and a group of obstetrics and gynecology physicians do not wish to advance their service, concentrate the hospital's resources on oncology and neurosciences.

One of the lessons that is repeatedly mentioned by hospital turnaround artists is that changes involving the medical staff should be made as soon as they are politically possible. Many administrators regret that they did not step up the recruitment of much needed physicians sooner or that so much time was exhausted catering to the medical staff's loners whose only interest is protecting their own secret gold mines.

Summary Comments

From the various chapters, from personal experience, and from a thorough review of the literature, it is apparent that in a hospital turnaround, the following principles hold true:

1. Quick action is often necessary; start early. The diagnosis of the organization should take place even before the CEO or manager arrives.

2. The CEO must often act more autocratically during the first part of a turnaround to take decisive, effective measures. During the corrective stage, there is often little time for collaboration.

3. Focus first on the expense side of the equation. Although expenses and revenue both should be examined, it is easier, in the short term, to affect expenses than revenues.

4. The approach should be multifaceted yet focused. It is important to determine the priority issues on both the expense and revenue sides of the equation and to move on them. Losers—losing managers and losing organizations—fail to concentrate, concentrate on the wrong subject, or concentrate on the right area but with inferior forces. Determine and clearly articulate the organization's priorities.

5. An employment contract and board support are absolutely essential. No CEO should be asked to turn around a hospital without some kind of employment contract. The administration cannot be expected to make the tough decisions if he or she is in constant fear of being unemployed and without compensation.

6. The CEO and the management team are expected to make tough decisions and must make them.

7. Communication can probably not be overdone. It must be frequent, factual, and positive. In addition, there is no substitute for the CEO being visible and directly communicating with all constituents.

8. The focus of the turnaround should be both internal and external. This is particularly true of public relations. Do not fail to ignore the external community in both market research and in communicating activities of the organization.

9. Cuts must be made as soon as possible and only once if possible. One does not cut off the tail of an animal one inch at a time, and one does not substantially cut staff more than once if it can be avoided. To limit cuts like this requires a clear definition of the target that is to be met.

10. There should be no holy cows; losers should get the ax.

11. Make cuts at the top first. It is important that management ranks be reduced before cutting employees at lower levels. Articulate and be able to defend the desired staff reductions clearly and often.

12. Success breeds success; start small if that luxury is available. Identify things that can be done to improve the organization and act on them.

13. Physicians must be part of the solution, or they will be part of the problem. Form a physician advisory group to work with the CEO in the turnaround.

14. Focus on short-term improvements while concurrently developing a long-range vision for the organization. A long-range plan is a must to an organization and must at least be done concurrently with the other turnaround processes.

15. Turnarounds are never complete. A turnaround is an ongoing process that, once initiated, must be sustained. Moreover, a successful turnaround must involve every major group in the hospital—board members, physicians, employees, and volunteers.

As this last truism indicates, turnarounds are dynamic and constantly require organizational renewal. The factors that contribute to organizational dry rot have already been mentioned and must receive both management and board attention. The ongoing monitoring of results and the modification of various systems to meet the needs of the ever-changing internal and external environment are absolutely essential. Indeed, to sustain a turnaround necessitates that form must follow function and not the reverse. A customer-oriented organization in today's health care climate is not the old authoritarian structure but an organization that has aggressive, bottom-up planning and accurate information and reporting systems.

Total quality management programs are being used in hospitals throughout the United States to ensure that turnarounds are sustained and that improvement continues. Such programs, combined with self-managing teams, can significantly improve hospital operations in the future. A self-managing team is responsible for recruiting, selecting, and scheduling assignments, and ensuring quality control. The supervisors are more consultants than actual supervisors.

It is probably true that most organizations are not suffering because they cannot solve their problems but because they cannot see their problems. Successful turnaround artists have acute listening skills and begin the turnaround process by conducting in-depth interviews with as many people as possible. They know that future operational changes must be based on sound information. Actions based on false assumptions are worse than no actions at all.

During the reduction phase, the turnaround artist distinguishes himself or herself from the amateur as much by the way he or she makes changes as by the kind of changes he or she makes. Anyone can downsize an organization, but the art comes in minimizing the trauma associated with reductions in services and staff and develop positive momentum in a climate of adversity. The turnaround artist is able to gain the respect of his or her superiors, subordinates, and others despite the harsh and rigorous nature of their work. They are leaders of the highest caliber.

The CEO and staff who attempt to turn around a hospital walk a fine line between moving aggressively, but not so aggressively that they derail the turnaround effort because it exceeds boundaries that are politically unacceptable to various hospital publics in general and the hospital board in particular. The successful turnaround artists have been able not only to identify the key issues that must be addressed but also to execute the necessary changes in such a way that they have preserved both their key staff members and themselves.

It is apparent that there are no quick fixes to turning a hospital around. Successful turnarounds are usually the result of long, arduous campaigns that are led by aggressive, tactically proficient CEOs. Although the CEO spark and lead such an effort, successful turnarounds require leadership at every level. Anyone can downsize an organization, but the art is to execute it in a way that minimizes the trauma and develops positive momentum in the face of adversity.

Notes

1. T. F. Moore and E. A. Simendinger, *Organizational Burnout in Healthcare Facilities: Strategies for Prevention and Change* (Rockville, MD: Aspen Publishers, 1985), 2.
2. M. Rindler, "The Successful Hospital Turnaround: It Starts with the Board," *Trustee*, December, 1987, 10.

3. R. Durham, "Defy the Odds," *Success*, November 1989, 18.
4. J. Gabarro, *The Dynamics of Taking Charge* (Boston, MA: Harvard Business School Press, 1985.
5. Ibid., 15.
6. Ibid., 20.
7. G. Goldstick, *Business Rx: How to Get in the Black and Stay There* (New York: John Wiley & Sons, 1988) 246–47.
8. J. Stewart, Jr., *Managing a Successful Business Turnaround* (New York: American Management Associates, 1984) 14–16 .
9. Goldstick, *Business Rx,* 142.
10. M. Rindler, *Managing a Hospital Turnaround: From Crisis to Profitability in Three Challenging Years* (Chicago: Pluribus Press, Inc., 1987), 36–37.
11. M. Rindler, *Managing a Hospital Turnaround,* 139.
12. Gabarro, *Dynamics of Taking Charge,* 51.
13. Rindler, *Managing a Hospital Turnaround,* 82.
14. D. Hunter, personal communication.

INDEX

LIST OF CONTRIBUTORS

Alethea O. Caldwell, FACHE, is the director of the Arizona Department of Health Services in Phoenix, Arizona. Previously, she was the president and chief executive officer of Ancilla Systems in Chicago. She received a master's degree from the University of California and a bachelor's degree from Pacific Union College.

Mark E. Celmer, FACHE, is the director and chief executive officer of DeGraff Memorial Hospital in North Tonawanda, New York. He received his undergraduate degree from Ithaca College in Ithaca, New York, and his master's degree in hospital administration from George Washington University in Washington, DC. In 1986 he was named Young Administrator of the Year by the American College of Healthcare Executives.

Richard J. Frenchie is president and chief executive officer of Geauga Hospital in Chardon, Ohio. He received his undergraduate degree from Cleveland State University and a master's degree from Baldwin-Wallace College.

John E. Friedlander is president and chief executive officer of Buffalo General Hospital in Buffalo, New York. He received his undergraduate degree from American International College in Springfield, Massachusetts, and his master's degree in health administration from Northeastern University in Boston, Massachusetts.

Charles H. Kachmarik, Jr., is a partner at Coopers and Lybrand in New York, New York. He received his undergraduate degree and master's degree from the State University of New York at Binghamton, New York.

Cheryl Minckler was the director of marketing at Valley Medical Center in Renton, Washington, at the time she collaborated on Chapter 2. She has since become a marketing consultant in Seattle, Washington. She received

231

a bachelor's degree in microbiology and immunology from the University of Washington and a master's degree in communications from the same university.

Joan E. Neuhaus is director of planning and marketing for Archbishop Bergan Mercy Hospital in Omaha, Nebraska. She received her bachelor's and master's degrees from Creighton University in Omaha.

William D. Nicely is president of St. Mary's Medical Center in Long Beach, California. Previously, he was president and chief executive officer of Archbishop Bergan Mercy Hospital in Omaha, Nebraska. He received his undergraduate degree from Ohio State University and his master's degree in hospital administration from Ohio State University.

Jeanne Bouxsein Parham is chief executive officer of Crawford Memorial Hospital in Van Buren, Arkansas. She received her undergraduate degree in hospital administration from the University of Illinois.

Daniel J. Rissing, FACHE, is president and chief executive officer of ProMedica Health System in Toledo, Ohio. Previously, he was president of the Hospital of St. Raphael in New Haven, Connecticut. From 1978 until 1988 he was president of Good Samaritan Medical Center in Zanesville, Ohio. He received his undergraduate degree from Indiana University and holds a master's degree in hospital administration from Xavier University.

Thomas H. Rockers is president and chief executive officer of Provenant Health Partners in Denver, Colorado. Previously, he was president and chief executive officer of Santa Rosa Health Care Corporation in San Antonio, Texas. He received his bachelor's degree from South Dakota State University and a master's degree in hospital administration from the University of Minnesota.

Richard D. Roodman is the administrator and chief executive officer of Valley Medical Center in Renton, Washington. He received his undergraduate degree from the University of Missouri and a master's degree in hospital administration from Washington University School of Medicine in St. Louis, Missouri.

Joseph M. Smith is vice president for operations at L.H.S. Management Company in Fargo, North Dakota, where he oversees the activities of a dozen hospitals in the United States. Previously, he was president of MidMichigan Regional Medical Center-Gladwin in Gladwin, Michigan. He holds a bachelor's degree from the University of Indiana and a master's degree from Central Michigan University.

R. Timothy Stack, FACHE, is president of Borgess Health Alliance in Kalamazoo, Michigan. He received a bachelor's degree from Betheny College and a master's degree from the Virginia Commonwealth University. In 1987 he received the Young Administrator of the Year Award from the American College of Healthcare Executives. He was president of the Southside Hospital of Pittsburgh, Pennsylvania, from 1982 until 1987.

ABOUT THE EDITORS

Terence F. Moore, M.B.A., M.H.A., is the president and CEO of MidMichigan Regional Health System, Midland, Michigan, which operates MidMichigan Regional Medical Center, MidMichigan Regional Medical Center–Clare, MidMichigan Regional Medical Center–Gladwin, MidMichigan Gladwin Pines Nursing Home, MidMichigan Stratford Pines Nursing Home, and five other subsidiaries. He holds a master's degree in hospital administration from the Washington University School of Medicine, St. Louis, Missouri, and bachelor of science and master of business administration degrees from Central Michigan University, where he has done additional graduate work in economics.

Mr. Moore is a fellow of the American College of Healthcare Executives. He is a past member of the board of the Michigan Hospital Association, treasurer of the board of the Michigan Molecular Institute, and past chairman of the board of the 23-member East Central Michigan Hospital Council. In 1986 he received the Regents Award for the state of Michigan from the American College of Healthcare Executives; in 1990 he received an honorary doctorate from Central Michigan University; and in 1992 he received the Meritorious Key Award from the Michigan Hospital Association.

He has published 60 articles and is the author of one book and the coauthor or coeditor of five others.

Earl A. Simendinger, Ph.D., is a professor of health education and health sciences at Central Michigan University. He is also the president of the Ivory Group, a management training and consultation firm in Mt. Pleasant, Michigan. Previously he held a joint adjunct associate professorship in the schools of medicine and engineering at Case Western Reserve University.

He has been a practicing hospital administrator for 19 years. His former positions include the presidency of St. Luke's Hospital, San Francisco, California, and a vice presidency at University Hospitals of Cleveland, Ohio.

Dr. Simendinger holds a doctoral degree in organizational behavior from Case Western Reserve University, a master's degree in health care administration from Washington University, St. Louis, Missouri, a master's degree in industrial engineering from Cleveland State University, and a bachelor's degree in business administration from Ashland College.

He is a fellow of the American College of Healthcare Executives and a member of the editorial review staff of both the *Journal of the American Medical Association* and *The Journal of Clinical Engineering*. He has published over 45 articles in health care management journals and has coauthored or coedited five books.

www.ingramcontent.com/pod-product-compliance
Lightning Source LLC
Chambersburg PA
CBHW021554210326
41599CB00010B/441